D0182579

OVERCOMING JEALOUSY

WINDY DRYDEN was born in London in 1950. He has
worked in psychotherapy and counselling for more than 30
years, and is the author or editor of over 160 books,
including *Letting Go of Anxiety and Depression* (Sheldon
Press, 2003) and *Assertiveness Step by Step* (written with
Daniel Constantinou, Sheldon Press, 2004). Dr Dryden is
Professor of Psychotherapeutic Studies at Goldsmiths
College, University of London.

Overcoming Common Problems Series

Selected titles
A full list of titles is available from Sheldon Press,
36 Causton Street, London SW1P 4ST, and on our website at
www.sheldonpress.co.uk

The Assertiveness Handbook
Mary Hartley

Assertiveness: Step by Step
Dr Windy Dryden and Daniel Constantinou

Body Language: What You Need to Know
David Cohen

Breaking Free
Carolyn Ainscough and Kay Toon

Calm Down
Paul Hauck

The Candida Diet Book
Karen Brody

Cataract: What You Need to Know
Mark Watts

The Chronic Fatigue Healing Diet
Christine Craggs-Hinton

Cider Vinegar
Margaret Hills

Comfort for Depression
Janet Horwood

The Complete Carer's Guide
Bridget McCall

The Confidence Book
Gordon Lamont

Confidence Works
Gladeana McMahon

Coping Successfully with Pain
Neville Shone

Coping Successfully with Panic Attacks
Shirley Trickett

Coping Successfully with Period Problems
Mary-Claire Mason

Coping Successfully with Prostate Cancer
Dr Tom Smith

Coping Successfully with Ulcerative Colitis
Peter Cartwright

Coping Successfully with Your Hiatus Hernia
Dr Tom Smith

Coping Successfully with Your Irritable Bowel
Rosemary Nicol

Coping with Age-related Memory Loss
Dr Tom Smith

Coping with Alopecia
Dr Nigel Hunt and Dr Sue McHale

Coping with Blushing
Dr Robert Edelmann

Coping with Bowel Cancer
Dr Tom Smith

Coping with Brain Injury
Maggie Rich

Coping with Candida
Shirley Trickett

Coping with Chemotherapy
Dr Terry Priestman

Coping with Childhood Allergies
Jill Eckersley

Coping with Childhood Asthma
Jill Eckersley

Coping with Chronic Fatigue
Trudie Chalder

Coping with Coeliac Disease
Karen Brody

Coping with Compulsive Eating
Ruth Searle

Coping with Diverticulitis
Peter Cartwright

Coping with Down's Syndrome
Fiona Marshall

Coping with Dyspraxia
Jill Eckersley

Coping with Eating Disorders and Body Image
Christine Craggs-Hinton

Coping with Endometriosis
Jo Mears

Coping with Family Stress
Mary-Claire Mason

Coping with Gout
Christine Craggs-Hinton

Coping with Hearing Loss
Christine Craggs-Hinton

Overcoming Common Problems Series

Overcoming Common Problems Series

Overcoming Common Problems

Overcoming Jealousy

Dr Windy Dryden

sheldon **PRESS**

First published in Great Britain in 1998

Sheldon Press
36 Causton Street
London SW1P 4ST

British Library Cataloguing in Publication Data
A catalogue record for this book is available
from the British Library

ISBN 978–0–85969–958–7

3 5 7 9 10 8 6 4

Typeset by Deltatype Ltd, Birkenhead, Merseyside
Printed in Great Britain by Ashford Colour Press

Produced on paper from sustainable forests

Contents

1
Introduction

In two of my previous books for Sheldon Press I made an important distinction between unhealthy and healthy negative emotions. Yes, your eyes haven't deceived you, I did use the phrase 'healthy negative emotions'. For some negative emotions are healthy. If you are facing, or think you are facing, a negative event, it is not healthy for you to feel good about the occurrence of this event, nor is it healthy for you to feel indifferent about it. Rather, it is healthy for you to feel bad about it. Feeling bad about a negative event helps you to think clearly about the event, to change it if it can be changed and to make a constructive adjustment to it if it can't be changed. By contrast, if you are unhealthily disturbed about the negative event this interferes with your ability to think clearly about it, you are less likely to change it in constructive ways if it can be changed, and if it can't be changed your adjustment is likely to be a poor one.

This means that in this book I will be talking about two different types of jealousy. The problem is that we do not have appropriate terms in the English language for healthy jealousy and unhealthy jealousy, so I will use these terms throughout this book even though they are not ideal.

Incidentally, there is a third type of jealousy – known as morbid jealousy – which falls outside the scope of this book. This is a psychiatric condition which requires psychiatric help. The main features of this type of jealousy are its delusional and obsessive nature. It takes over your life and you can't get any peace. You are convinced that your partner is constantly interested in other members of the opposite sex and you are sure that you have clear-cut evidence to back up your claims. You cannot get these thoughts out of your mind and it literally dominates your waking moments and invades your dreams. If you think that you suffer from morbid jealousy, please consult your doctor as soon as possible.

INTRODUCTION
The ABC framework

The approach to counselling that I practise is known as Rational Emotive Behaviour Therapy (REBT). It was founded in 1955 by Albert Ellis, an American clinical psychologist, whose voluminous writings have helped REBT to become a well-known and popular therapy over forty years later. REBT has a simple ABC framework which I will now discuss. You will be able to use this framework to understand your experiences of unhealthy jealousy and later to change these disturbed feelings.

A

In the ABC framework, A stands for activating event. This is an event which represents the beginning of an emotional episode, in this case jealousy. Now, As can either represent actual events or inferences. This is a very important distinction which you need to grasp if you are to understand jealousy and, in particular, the difference between healthy and unhealthy jealousy.

Let me begin my discussion by defining an inference. An inference is a hunch about reality that goes beyond the information available to you. As such, an inference may be accurate or inaccurate. You don't know which is the case until you get more information. Often, you cannot get the information you need to tell for certain whether or not an inference is correct, and in such cases you need to go for what is probably the case rather than what is definitely the case.

Let me give you a few examples of the differences between actual events and inferences. In doing so, I will discuss an instance where a person accepts an inference as a fact when this is probably warranted and a case where a person accepts an inference as a fact when this is probably not warranted.

Terry and Gina, a young married couple, are at a party and Terry goes off to get Gina a drink. When he returns, Gina is talking to another man and is sharing a joke with him. Terry notes that this is happening and thinks to himself (or infers) that Gina is sharing a joke with the man, and thinks nothing more of it.

2

Simon and Theresa, who are also a young married couple, are at the same party and exactly the same thing happens. Simon goes off to get Theresa a drink, and when he returns Theresa is talking to another man and is sharing a joke with him. Simon notes that this is happening and thinks to himself that Theresa wants to get off with the other man. Simon's thought that Theresa wants to get off with the other man is an inference that goes beyond the information available to Simon. Is Simon's inference probably accurate or probably inaccurate? Based just on the information that is immediately available to Simon, this inference is probably inaccurate because all Simon knows is that Theresa is laughing with the man. But let us suppose that Theresa has a long history of going off with men at parties and that this often starts with her laughing at a man's jokes. In this case, Simon's inference is probably accurate because it is based on a fact about Theresa's behaviour at parties. If, however, Theresa has no such history, then Simon's inference that she wants to go off with this particular man is probably inaccurate.

As I will show you later, when you are unhealthily jealous you tend to make inferences that your partner is interested in another person in the absence of corroborating evidence. What is more, you treat such inferences as incontrovertible facts and often twist information to fit in with these 'facts'. The reasons why you do this will soon become apparent.

B

In the ABC framework, B stands for beliefs. The theory of Rational Emotive Behaviour Therapy distinguishes between two different types of beliefs: rational and irrational beliefs. Rational beliefs have five major characteristics. They are:

1 flexible and non-extreme;
2 conducive to mental health;
3 helpful to the person as he strives towards his goals;

4 realistic or true;
5 logical or sensible.

REBT theory argues that there are four major rational beliefs. These are known as:

1 Full preferences (e.g. 'I want my partner to be only interested in me, but it is not essential that she is').
2 Anti-awfulizing (e.g. 'It would be very bad if my partner was interested in someone else, but it wouldn't be the end of the world').
3 Low frustration tolerance (e.g. 'It would be difficult for me to tolerate it if my partner was interested in someone else, but I could bear it').
4 Acceptance. There are two types of acceptance beliefs: self-acceptance (e.g. 'If my partner was interested in someone else it would not prove that I was less worthy. My worth is constant and does not go up and down according to whether or not my partner is interested in someone else') and other-acceptance (e.g. 'If my partner is interested in someone else he would not be a rotten person. Rather, he would be a fallible human being who would be doing what in my view is the wrong thing').

Irrational beliefs also have five major characteristics. They are:

1 rigid and extreme;
2 conducive to psychological disturbance;
3 unhelpful to the person as he strives towards his goals;
4 unrealistic or false;
5 illogical or nonsensical.

REBT theory argues that there are four major irrational beliefs. These are known as:

1 Musts or demands (e.g. 'My partner must only be interested in me').

2 Awfulizing (e.g. 'It would be terrible if my partner was interested in someone else').
3 Low frustration tolerance (e.g. 'I couldn't bear it if my partner was interested in someone else').
4 Depreciation. There are two types of depreciation beliefs: self-depreciation (e.g. 'If my partner was interested in someone else it would prove that I was less worthy') and other-depreciation (e.g. 'If my partner was interested in someone else it would prove that he was a rotten person').

C

In the ABC framework, C stands for consequences of the beliefs at B that you hold about the activating events you focus on at A. There are three types of consequences: emotional consequences, behavioural consequences and thinking consequences.

Emotional consequences

When you hold a set of rational beliefs about a negative activating agent then you will experience a healthy negative emotion. Thus, if you think that your partner is interested in somebody else, and you prefer, but do not demand, that this doesn't happen, then you will experience healthy jealousy, whereas when you hold a set of irrational beliefs about a negative activating event then you will experience an unhealthy negative emotion. Thus, if you think that your partner is interested in someone else and you demand that this must not happen, then you will experience unhealthy jealousy.

Behavioural consequences

When you hold a set of rational beliefs about a negative activating event then you will either act in a functional way or you will feel like acting in such a manner (this urge to act is known as an action tendency). Thus, if you think that your partner is interested in somebody else and you prefer, but do not demand, that this doesn't happen, then you will tell your partner about your concerns and discuss the issue with him in an assertive manner.

However, if you hold a set of irrational beliefs about a negative activating event then you will either act in a dysfunctional way or you will feel like acting in such a manner. Thus, if you think that your partner is interested in someone else and you demand that this doesn't happen, then you will accuse him of this and attempt to restrict his movements, for example.

Thinking consequences

When you hold a set of rational beliefs about a negative activating event then your thinking will be constructive and realistic. Thus, if you think that your partner is interested in somebody else and you prefer, but do not demand, that this doesn't happen, then you will look for evidence that both supports and contradicts your hypothesis. You will be able to stand back and evaluate all of this evidence in an objective manner and arrive at a conclusion which best fits the available data. If you conclude that your partner is interested in the other person, then you will consider this in a broad context. Thus, if your relationship with your partner is basically good and he does not regularly show interest in other women, then you will judge that the threat to your relationship is small. However, if your relationship with your partner is not good and he regularly shows interest in other women, then you may realistically conclude that the threat to your relationship is greater and that your partner may leave you, particularly if he shows great interest in the other woman.

On the other hand, when you hold a set of irrational beliefs about a negative activating event then your thinking will be unconstructive and unrealistic. If you think that your partner is interested in somebody else and you demand that this must not happen, then you will look for evidence that supports your view and edit out or explain away evidence that contradicts your view. Thus, you will not tend to stand back and evaluate all of the evidence that is available to you; if you do, you will not do so in an objective manner, and so you will not arrive at a conclusion which best fits the available data. Following your strongly held conviction that your partner is definitely interested in the other person, you will not consider this in a broad context. Thus, you will tend to think that your partner will leave you for the other woman whether or not you have a good relationship with him and whether or not he regularly shows interest in other women.

6

Beliefs affect inferences

So far, I have presented the ABC framework as if the three elements are separate. However, in reality they are not. In fact, the ABC elements often interact in highly complex ways. While full coverage of the complex interactions among As, Bs and Cs lies outside the scope of this book, I will discuss one such interaction as it is very important to a full understanding of jealousy, and in particular unhealthy jealousy.

It is important for you to understand that when you hold one or more irrational beliefs, especially when you have held these for a long time, you bring these irrational beliefs to events that relate to your relationship with your partner. This means that your irrational beliefs make you particularly prone to make jealousy-related inferences. Let me give you an example of this.

Jeremy believed that whoever he went out with had to be only interested in him. If his girlfriend of the moment showed any interest in another man, even when this was clearly only a mark of politeness, then this led Jeremy to think that he was inferior to that person. Jeremy was handsome and women found him very charming; he had little trouble finding girlfriends. However, he had enormous trouble sustaining these relationships. Why? Because Jeremy brought his irrational belief to situations where his girlfriend of the moment came into contact with other men of her age. When this happened, Jeremy's irrational belief led him to infer that his girlfriend was interested romantically and sexually in the other man and that if she spent more than a few minutes talking to him then the two of them would soon make plans to meet and an affair between them would ensue. No matter how many times Jeremy was reassured by his various girlfriends that they were only being sociable and had not the slightest interest in the men they were talking to, Jeremy still made the same inference. Indeed, as long as Jeremy believed that his girlfriend of the moment must only be interested in him, this belief would invariably lead him to infer that the interest she showed in other men couldn't just be polite sociability, but had to be of a romantic and sexual nature. In addition, since Jeremy believed himself to be inferior to other men, he tended to see these other men as superior to him and consequently more attractive and more interesting to his girlfriends.

As I will discuss presently, it wasn't these inferences and the beliefs that spawned them which were alone responsible for the breakdown of virtually all of Jeremy's relationships. Rather, it was the way Jeremy acted towards his girlfriends that led them to leave him. Eventually, all of them concluded that they were unprepared to put up with Jeremy's endless interrogations and unreasonable restrictions on whom they could and could not speak to. However, Jeremy would not have behaved in such relationship-defeating ways, nor inferred that his relationships were constantly under threat, if he had not held the irrational belief that his girlfriend must not show any interest in other men, and that if she did this would prove that he was inferior.

So far in this opening chapter I have introduced you to the basic ABC framework that is the hallmark of Rational Emotive Behaviour Therapy. This framework is particularly useful for analysing and understanding why you experience unhealthy jealousy in specific situations. If you are particularly prone to experiencing this unhealthy emotion, you can also use the ABC framework to understand why this is so.

However, you have probably not bought this book just to understand unhealthy jealousy. You are probably interested in how to overcome this unhealthy emotion when it becomes problematic for you. To help you to do this, you first have to understand REBT's full model of personal change. This comprehensive model begins with the ABC elements that I have already discussed. After all, you cannot really change something before you have understood it. And, as I have stressed, the ABC framework is designed to provide you with an overall picture of what is going on when you experience unhealthy jealousy. But to change this unhealthy emotion you will have to understand and implement four other steps. These steps are known as the DEFG part of the comprehensive REBT model of personal change. I will, of course, discuss in detail how you can overcome unhealthy jealousy later in the book (see Chapters 4 and

5). What I will do here is to give you a brief overall understanding of the DEFG part of the ABCDEFG model. I will begin by discussing G.

G

In the ABCDEFG framework, G stands for goals. If you are troubled by feelings of unhealthy jealousy and you wish to overcome these feelings, you need to have a clear idea of what you would be prepared to experience instead, given the actual existence of the activating event at A in the framework. After all, if your partner is interested in someone else and you are experiencing unhealthy jealousy, is it realistic for you to set as your goal that you want to be pleased about this? Don't forget that you would still prefer to have the exclusive interest of your partner. What is wrong with feeling healthily jealous, which means that you want to have an exclusive relationship with your partner even though you do not demand it? In my view there is nothing wrong with feeling healthily jealous – it may even discourage you in the long run from taking your partner for granted. It is not only important to set a goal when you recognize that you are experiencing an unhealthy negative emotion like unhealthy jealousy, it is also important to set a goal which will help you in the long run and which is appropriate to the negative activating event that you are actually confronted with or that you think that you are confronted with. Finally, setting healthy goals to which you are committed motivates you to do the work that you need to do in the DEF part of the personal change process.

D

In the ABCDEFG framework, D stands for disputing the irrational beliefs that account for your feelings of unhealthy jealousy. As I will discuss in greater detail later in this book, disputing your irrational beliefs involves asking yourself whether your irrational beliefs are true or false, logical or illogical and helpful or unhelpful. As I will show you later, irrational beliefs are in general false, illogical and unhelpful. Disputing also involves you asking yourself whether your alternative rational beliefs are true or false, logical or illogical and helpful or unhelpful. Again, as I will discuss in fuller detail in due course, rational beliefs are, in general, true, logical and helpful.

E

In the ABCDEFG framework, E stands for the effects of the disputing techniques you have employed in the previous step. If you have effectively disputed your irrational beliefs and have understood that they are false, illogical and unhelpful and that your alternative rational beliefs are true, logical and helpful then you will begin to notice that: your feelings begin to change from unhealthy negative emotions to healthy negative emotions; you begin to act more functionally; and your subsequent thinking becomes more objective, realistic and balanced.

On the other hand, if your feelings, behaviour and subsequent thinking do not change then this tells you that you need to return to the previous disputing stage and question your irrational and rational beliefs again.

F

In the ABCDEFG framework, F stands for facilitating change. In order to bring about a meaningful change in your emotions, behaviour and subsequent thinking, then you need to take the following steps and implement them again and again:

1 Repeatedly question your irrational and rational beliefs and show yourself that the former are false, illogical and unhelpful and the latter are true, sensible and helpful. The more arguments you can develop during this stage the better, and the more forceful and energetically you can do this the better.
2 Resolve to act in ways that are consistent with your rational beliefs and that are inconsistent with your irrational beliefs. If you successfully dispute the irrational beliefs that underpin your unhealthy jealousy, but you continue to act in ways that are consistent with your jealous feelings, you will only succeed in nullifying any benefits that you gained from the disputing stage. Changing your behaviour may well involve acting against your well-rehearsed unhealthy jealous behaviour, but this is what you need to do if you are to facilitate a healthy personal change.

3 Question the inferences that you easily make when you feel unhealthily jealous. Again, if you allow yourself to treat these distorted inferences as facts then you will elaborate them, and doing so will again tend to nullify the benefits that you gained from the disputing stage.

If you are successful in the facilitating change stage then you will have been successful at reaching your goals at G in the change framework.

In conclusion, in this chapter I distinguished between healthy and unhealthy jealousy and outlined the ABCDEFG framework that details the steps you need to take to overcome your feelings of unhealthy jealousy. In the next chapter, I will focus on unhealthy jealousy and discuss in detail the factors that underpin this destructive emotion.

2

The ABCs of Unhealthy Jealousy

In this chapter, I will consider what people tend to be unhealthily jealous about and discuss the attitudes that underpin unhealthy jealousy. I will also consider what people tend to do and think when they experience unhealthy jealousy, and show how these forms of behaviour and thinking serve to maintain unhealthy jealousy. I will use Rational Emotive Behaviour Therapy's ABC framework, introduced in the opening chapter, as a way of structuring this material.

As you read this chapter I want you to remember a point that I stressed in the first chapter, that there are two main types of jealousy: unhealthy jealousy and healthy jealousy. In this chapter, I will focus on unhealthy jealousy and will discuss healthy jealousy in the following chapter.

What we feel unhealthily jealous about

I have practised as a counsellor and psychotherapist for approaching twenty-five years and in that time I have had many clients who have sought help for their unhealthy jealousy. In virtually all cases their unhealthy jealousy concerned one event: they were convinced that there existed a serious threat to the relationship that they had with a significant other. Now, in this book I will concentrate on romantic jealousy, i.e. the jealousy that people experience when they are romantically involved with another person. However, as I will soon show, jealousy can also be experienced in non-romantic relationships.

Here is a typical example of unhealthy romantic jealousy.

Miriam had been going out with Jack for about a month when they were invited to a party. On her return from the lavatory, Miriam saw Jack dancing with another woman and immediately felt unhealthily jealous. What was it to do with this seemingly innocuous situation that Miriam felt unhealthily jealous about? Why wasn't she pleased that Jack seemed to be enjoying himself, which after all is the prime purpose of going to a party? The answer to these questions is that Miriam viewed Jack dancing with the other woman and appearing to enjoy himself as a threat to her relationship with him.

There you have it. What you are most likely to feel unhealthily jealous about is the threat posed by a third person to your relationship with someone important to you. The essential ingredients in a situation in which you experience unhealthy jealousy are as follows:

- you
- a person who is important to you, with whom you are in some kind of relationship
- another person who, in your mind, poses a threat to that relationship.

Let me take a closer look at these elements. Perhaps the most important aspect of any jealousy scenario is the triangular nature of the situation, i.e. three people are involved. This feature distinguishes jealousy from envy. You can be envious of another person without a third person being involved, whereas the three-person situation is a defining characteristic of jealousy.

The second feature of a jealousy scenario that I wish to highlight is that you believe you have some kind of relationship with someone you deem to be significant to you. Now, in most jealousy scenarios the relationship that you have with the other person is a real one. However, in other jealousy scenarios, albeit in a minority of cases, the relationship exists in your head. In other words, you think that you have a relationship with the other person even though in reality you do not.

For example, Gina had very strong feelings for John and thought that he was interested in her even though the two of them had never been out together. When Gina discovered that John had started going out with Janice, Gina felt strong feelings of unhealthy jealousy because she saw Janice as a threat to the relationship that she thought she had with John.

So far I have discussed unhealthy romantic jealousy. However, unhealthy jealousy can exist in non-romantic, non-sexual relationships as well.

For example, Roberta was a talented swimmer and the apple of her coach's eye. Everybody recognized that Roberta was her coach's favourite protégée and Roberta herself basked in his attention. Then one day a younger girl joined the swimming team; she had an exceptional talent and immediately the coach paid her even more attention than he paid to Roberta. Roberta's response was to feel very unhealthily jealous about their relationship because she considered the new girl to be a threat to the relationship that she had with her coach.

Unhealthy jealousy is often experienced by young children when a new baby arrives on the scene.

For example, Harry was three when his baby sister, Jessica, was born. Until that time, Harry had enjoyed the exclusive love and attention of his devoted parents. Now, Jessica's arrival posed a threat to Harry's exclusive relationship with his parents and he responded with unhealthy jealousy by hitting his sister and misbehaving whenever his parents paid attention to Jessica and neglected him. So you see, unhealthy jealousy can be experienced in the context of non-romantic, non-sexual relationships and can be experienced quite early in life.

The nature of the threat in unhealthy jealousy

When you regard a third person as a threat to your relationship, what is the nature of this threat? In my view the nature of this threat is fourfold.

14

1 You regard the other person as someone who will replace you in the affections of your partner and think that your partner will leave you for the other person.
2 You think that your partner finds the other person more attractive than you and, while you don't think that she will go off with the other person, you consider that you will be displaced as the most important person in her life. Here, while you are not threatened by your partner's interest in the other person, you are threatened by the fact (in your mind) that you will no longer be the most important person in her life, that she gives a higher priority to the other person than she does to you.
3 It is important to you that your partner is only interested in you and you are threatened by any interest that she shows in another person. Here, while exclusivity is important to you, you do not necessarily think that your partner is going to leave you.
4 It is important that no-one shows any interest in your partner, and you are threatened by any interest that another person shows in your partner. Here, your focus is on the other person rather than on your partner.

Real and inferred events in unhealthy jealousy

As I mentioned in Chapter 1, you can experience unhealthy jealousy about an actual threat to your relationship with your partner, for example, or about a threat which you think exists, but which in reality doesn't. In the latter case, you infer the existence of a threat to your relationship and, rather than regarding this as a hypothesis about reality, you regard it as a fact and react accordingly.

Let me give you an example of someone who felt unhealthily jealous about inferred threats to his relationship.

Daniel had been going out with Linda for about two months and they had been getting on famously. Although they had not made a formal agreement to do so, they developed the habit of speaking to one another every day on the telephone. One day, Daniel rang Linda and, as she was not in, left a message on her answer machine to the effect that she should call him back when she got in. As luck would have it, Linda's answer machine was faulty and did not record Daniel's message. When Linda got home after an evening out with her two girlfriends she was dog tired and, having established that there were no messages on her answer machine, turned the ringer of the phone off and went to bed. Daniel waited until midnight and then rang Linda, but only got through to her answer machine. At this point Daniel became convinced that Linda had lied to him and in fact had not gone out with her girlfriends, but had gone out with another man with whom she was staying the night. Every time Daniel got through to Linda's answer machine, as he did on numerous occasions that night, his conviction that she was spending the night with another man deepened. After snatching a few hours of fitful sleep, Daniel woke in the morning completely convinced that Linda had spent the night with another man.

Note a number of important things about this incident. First, the actual situation facing Daniel at A in the ABC framework was that Linda did not return the message that he thought he had left on her answer machine. His inference about this situation was that she had spent the night with another man. Daniel would not have felt unhealthily jealous if he had stuck with the facts of the situation or if he had formed an inference based on what he knew about Linda: that she had shown herself to be trustworthy and that there would be a good reason for her not returning his message. However, the fact was that Daniel did infer from the information available to him that Linda had spent the night with another man, and this is what he was unhealthily jealous about.

People who regularly experience unhealthy jealousy do tend to make inferences at A in the ABC framework in which they see their relationship threatened by a third person. I will explain why this is the case presently.

The past, present and future in unhealthy jealousy

So far, I have discussed unhealthy jealousy that is experienced about events that exist (or are deemed by you to exist) in the present and which you regard as posing some kind of threat to your relationship. Indeed, present-related unhealthy jealousy, as it might be called, is probably the most common form of unhealthy jealousy. However, it is possible to feel unhealthily jealous about past events and even about events that have not happened yet.

Here is an example of past-related unhealthy jealousy.

> Michael had been dating Cheryl for about a year and had not experienced unhealthy jealousy in all this time. Then, he discovered some old photos where Cheryl was intimately kissing another man whom she had dated for a few months. From that point Michael became very unhealthily jealous about the relationship that Cheryl had had with the man in the photograph. Michael was not unhealthily jealous about present threats to his relationship with Cheryl, just about this past threat.

You may be wondering how a past relationship can be seen as a threat to a current relationship. After all, that relationship has ended and in all probability your partner will never see that other person again. However, in the case of Michael, what was threatening to him was the thought that Cheryl had found the other man more attractive than him, and wished that she was with him rather than with Michael. In another case, Keith was unhealthily jealous of Martha's previous relationships because he insisted that he be the only man in her life ever. The author Julian Barnes has written a compelling novel entitled *Before She Met Me* (Jonathan Cape, 1992) which details the tragic consequences of past-related unhealthy jealousy and is worth reading.

> In an example of future-related unhealthy jealousy, Maria, a 50-year-old woman, married Stephen, who was 26 years old. Maria was preoccupied with unhealthy jealous thoughts about women that Stephen might find more attractive than her when, at some time in the future, he started to view her as an old woman. Interestingly, Maria was not unhealthily jealous about women that Stephen might meet in the present because she was sure that he found her attractive. It was only when Maria thought about a time in the future when Stephen ceased to find her attractive that she became unhealthily jealous.

17

It is important to note that, in both past-related unhealthy jealousy and future-related unhealthy jealousy, the person who is unhealthily jealous perceives a threat to his or her relationship. In this important respect these forms of unhealthy jealousy are similar to present-related unhealthy jealousy where the threat to one's relationship is more apparent.

Why we feel unhealthily jealous

So far I have discussed what people feel unhealthily jealous about, namely an actual or, more frequently, a perceived threat to an important relationship. However, it is important for you to understand that what we feel unhealthily jealous about is not the same issue as why we feel unhealthily jealous. Let me use the ABC part of the ABCDEFG framework to explain what I mean.

If you recall, in Chapter 1 I explained that A stands for an activating event (actual or inferred), B stands for your beliefs about this activating event and C stands for the emotional, behavioural and thinking consequences of your beliefs about A. Applying the ABC part of the overall framework, this means that when you experience unhealthy jealousy (at C) about an actual or perceived threat to your relationship (at A) you experience this unhealthy reaction not because of the threat itself but because of the beliefs that you hold about this threat.

In other words, A does not determine C on its own. Rather, your beliefs about A determine C. This does not mean, of course, that A is irrelevant. Far from it. If you did not infer that a threat to your relationship existed then you wouldn't experience unhealthy jealousy (or healthy jealousy, come to that, as I will show you in the next chapter). What it means is that the existence of a threat to your relationship on its own does not account for your experience of unhealthy jealousy. To experience unhealthy jealousy, you have to hold a set of irrational beliefs about that threat.

Let me sum up my position on this point.

1 Facing (or thinking that you face) a threat to your relationship is a

necessary condition for unhealthy jealousy to be experienced, but it is not sufficient for this emotional state to be experienced.

2 Facing (or thinking that you face) a threat to your relationship plus holding a set of irrational beliefs are necessary and sufficient conditions for unhealthy jealousy to be experienced.

Having argued that the determining factor in unhealthy jealousy is the set of irrational beliefs about the threat that you face (or think that you face) to your relationship, let me consider in greater detail the nature of these irrational beliefs. You will recall from Chapter 1 that REBT emphasizes four such beliefs: rigid demands; awfulizing beliefs; low frustration tolerance (LFT) beliefs; and depreciation beliefs, where the person depreciates him or herself, other people and/or life conditions. While these four irrational beliefs are interlinked, I will deal with them one at a time. I will begin with rigid demands because Albert Ellis, the founder of Rational Emotive Behaviour Therapy, argues that if irrational beliefs are at the heart of psychological disturbance including unhealthy jealousy, then rigid demands are at its very core.

Rigid demands

Holding rigid demands is at the very core of a variety of emotional problems and this is certainly the case in unhealthy jealousy. Rigid demands tend to be dogmatic versions of perfectly legitimate and healthy full preferences (which I will discuss further in Chapter 3). In REBT, we normally do not question full preferences because they are flexible and allow for one's desires and wants not being met, but we do question rigid demands because, as I will now show you, they are dogmatic and tyrannical.

Let me give you several examples of the main rigid demands that underpin unhealthy jealousy.

'My partner must only be interested in me.'

'My partner is allowed to find other people attractive, but she must find me more attractive than anyone else.'

'I must be the only person that my partner has ever been in love with.'

'I must know for certain that my partner is not in the company of other men.'

'I must know for certain that my partner is not thinking about anyone of the opposite sex.'

'My partner must not engage in activities with members of the opposite sex that absolutely should be exclusive to our relationship.'

'No other woman must show interest in my partner.'

Awfulizing beliefs

Awfulizing beliefs are extreme evaluations of badness which do not allow for anything to be worse and stem, according to Albert Ellis, from one's rigid demands. I will go over the list that I presented when discussing rigid demands and show how awfulizing beliefs fit into the picture.

'My partner must be only interested in me and it would be terrible if she were interested in someone else.'

'My partner is allowed to find other people attractive, but she must find me more attractive than anyone else. It would be terrible if she found someone more attractive than me.'

'I must be the only person that my partner has ever been in love with, and it would be horrible if I weren't.'

'I must know for certain that my partner is not in the company of other men, and it would be awful if I didn't.'

'I must know for certain that my partner is not thinking about anyone of the opposite sex, and it would be terrible if I didn't have such certainty.'

'My partner must not engage in activities with members of the opposite sex that absolutely should be exclusive to our relationship. It would be the end of the world if I discovered that he has been doing these things with other women.'

20

'No other woman must show interest in my partner, and it would be horrendous if one did.'

Low frustration tolerance (LFT) beliefs

LFT beliefs indicate that the person holding them believes that he is unable to tolerate a particular event. Again, Ellis argues that LFT beliefs stem from rigid demands, as shown in the following:

'My partner must be only interested in me and it is unbearable if she is not.'

'My partner is allowed to find other people attractive, but she must find me more attractive than anyone else. I couldn't bear it if she found someone else more attractive than me.'

'I must be the only person that my partner has ever been in love with. If she had been in love before, I couldn't tolerate that.'

'I must know for certain that my partner is not in the company of other men, and I can't bear the uncertainty of not knowing.'

'I must know for certain that my partner is not thinking about anyone of the opposite sex. Not knowing that he is not is intolerable to me.'

'My partner must not engage in activities with members of the opposite sex that absolutely should be exclusive to our relationship. If she did engage in such activities with other men, I couldn't stand it.'

'No other woman must show interest in my partner. I couldn't put up with such a situation.'

Depreciation beliefs

Depreciation beliefs involve giving oneself and other people a global negative rating. Once again, according to Ellis, depreciation beliefs stem from rigid demands (as shown below) although not all rigid beliefs lead to depreciation beliefs.

'My partner must be only interested in me and if she is not this proves that I am worthless.'

'My partner is allowed to find other people attractive, but she must find me more attractive than anyone else. If she finds someone else more attractive than me this proves that I am less worthy than the other person.'

'I must be the only person that my partner has ever been in love with. If not, this proves that I am not as lovable as the other person.'

'My partner must not engage in activities with members of the opposite sex that absolutely should be exclusive to our relationship. If this does happen then I will be exposed to other people as a fool.'

'No other woman must show interest in my partner. If she does, she is a bitch.'

To sum up, according to this analysis threats to our relationships (real or inferred) posed by third persons do not, on their own, explain why we feel unhealthy jealousy. Rather, we feel unhealthy jealousy because we hold one or more irrational beliefs about such threats.

Unhealthy jealousy and other unhealthy negative emotions

So far I have viewed unhealthy jealousy as an emotion in its own right. Using the ABC part of the ABCDEFG framework I have shown the following:

A = real or inferred threat to our relationship posed by a third person

B = irrational beliefs (rigid demands, awfulizing beliefs, LFT beliefs, depreciation beliefs)

C = unhealthy jealousy.

There is another view in the field of psychology, however, that states that unhealthy jealousy is not a single emotion. Rather, it is a complex mixture of different emotions. I will now take this view and discuss those unhealthy negative emotions which make up unhealthy jealousy. In doing so, I will discuss anxiety, anger, hurt, depression and shame, since these seem to be the major emotions that comprise jealousy.

Anxiety

If you experience unhealthy jealousy, the chances are that you will be anxious much of the time. You will be constantly vigilant for signs that your partner may be interested in someone else or that someone else may be interested in your partner and, as I will soon discuss, you tend to read threat into even the most innocent interchanges between your partner and members of the opposite sex. As such, you find it difficult to relax when you are with your partner in mixed company, because you are constantly analysing who says what to whom and what they meant by it. You also find it difficult to relax when you are not in the company of your partner because you are constantly wondering who he is talking to and what they are saying.

When unhealthy jealousy becomes a real problem for you (and your partner, since, almost by definition, when you suffer from unhealthy jealousy, your partner does too), you cannot even relax when you are on your own with your partner. Consider what life would be like if you were in Marion's shoes.

As a result of Marion's unhealthy jealousy she and her husband, Vic, spent little time with other people (because Marion believed that she couldn't bear the thought of Vic looking at and talking to other women) and Vic spent very little time apart from Marion (becaused Marion believed that she couldn't bear the thought of Vic being in the same room as other women). However, even being together with Vic in their own home did not lessen Marion's anxiety. For example, she was constantly nervous while they were both watching the television in case an attractive female would appear on the TV screen, and she was even anxious while they were both reading separate books in case Vic came across a sexy scene in his book and wished that he was with the woman in the novel rather than with her. She was anxious when they were doing nothing in case Vic started thinking about an attractive woman, and she was anxious about going to bed in case Vic would dream of another women. Even when they made love, she couldn't relax. Why? You've guessed it; because she was scared that Vic was thinking of making love to another woman when he was making love to her.

Marion's sad plight shows quite clearly that when you are unhealthily jealous, anxiety is virtually your constant companion. The anxiety that forms a part of the unhealthy jealousy complex of emotions has three major components:

1 A threat (real or perceived) to what is important to you.
2 A dogmatic insistence that this threat must not exist.
3 The idea that it would be terrible if the threat materialized.

Unhealthy anger

Anger is another emotion that is often experienced by people who feel unhealthy jealousy frequently. I distinguish between healthy anger (where you attempt to deal with situations you don't like in ways that demonstrate your respect for the other person) and unhealthy anger (where you try to assert your will in ways that condemn the other person). You will not be surprised to learn that the kind of anger that frequently accompanies unhealthy jealousy is the unhealthy kind.

People who frequently experience unhealthy jealousy often have rules that they believe other people, and in particular their partners, have to live by. It is the demand that the other has to abide by these rules that is at the core of unhealthy anger here. Here is a typical example.

Bernadette and Paul would sometimes go down to their local pub for a few drinks. Bernadette, who had a long-standing problem with unhealthy jealousy, had a rule which stated that it was wrong for Paul to look at other women in the pub when he was with her. This rule was bad enough, but it was made far worse by Bernadette's insistence that Paul had to abide by it, and when she thought that he had violated this rule she would subject him to a tirade of verbal abuse mixed with accusations thinly disguised as questions.

'How dare you ogle that woman when you know I don't like it! I told you last time we were out that I find it offensive. Why are you doing this to me? You really are a bastard, Paul. I know you'd rather be with her than me. But why do you have to make it so obvious?'

This is the kind of abuse that people who have a problem with unhealthy jealousy heap on their partners. The unhealthy anger that forms a part of the unhealthy jealousy complex of emotions has three major components:

1 A rule of conduct for the partner to follow. This rule either prescribes behaviour (i.e. indicates the behaviour the partner is expected to follow) or prohibits behaviour (i.e. indicates the behaviour that the partner is expected to refrain from).
2 A dogmatic insistence that the partner absolutely must abide by this rule.
3 The expression of a condemnatory attitude when the partner breaks the rule.

Hurt

When hurt is a feature of unhealthy jealousy, you think that your partner has betrayed you and you consider that you have done nothing to deserve this unfair treatment. Hurt often leads to sulking, and in my clinical experience people who frequently experience unhealthy jealousy also oscillate between overt expressions of anger and some form of sulking behaviour.

As soon as Peter and June got married, Peter began to show signs of unhealthy jealousy. Peter was unemployed while June had a

25

well-paid professional job, a situation which fuelled Peter's insecurity and his unhealthy jealousy. Because he had a lot of time on his hands, Peter spent long periods of time on his own, thinking of all the men at her work that June was flirting with. When June came home, Peter interrogated June concerning what she did that day and who she spoke to. After a while, June refused to give Peter a blow-by-blow account of her interacting, a situation to which Peter responded with anger and then hurt. Peter felt hurt because he considered June's refusal to tell him about her day as an undeserved betrayal of trust. When this happened, Peter became sullen and would not talk to June for hours.

The feelings of hurt that form a part of the unhealthy jealousy complex of emotions have three major components:

1   The idea that your partner has betrayed you and that you do not deserve this treatment.
2   A dogmatic insistence that your partner absolutely should not have done this.
3   A 'poor me' attitude.

Depression

When depression is a feature of unhealthy jealousy, you tend to focus on the idea that you are basically an unworthy, unlovable person, and therefore your partner is bound to want to go off with the first person that she finds more attractive and more interesting than you. In your mind this is the very next reasonably presentable man that she comes into contact with.

Another idea that is associated with the depressive part of the unhealthy jealousy experience relates to the idea that you will always be unhealthily jealous and thus will always have difficult relationships with the opposite sex, which will be terrible.

The feelings of depression that form a part of the unhealthy jealousy complex of emotions have three major components:

1   The inference that you are bound to lose your partner to someone else.

2 The belief that this must not happen, even though a part of you recognizes that it is inevitable.
3 The belief that you are worthless, an idea which convinces you that you are bound to lose this partner and any others that you may have in the future and which is reinforced if you do, in fact, lose your partner.

Shame

When shame is a feature of unhealthy jealousy, you focus on what any threat to your relationship reveals about you to others. Shame involves you viewing yourself as a diminished person, a defective person or a disgraced person. In jealousy-related shame you are preoccupied with the idea that your partner will make you appear foolish or a laughing stock in the eyes of others, which would strengthen your own idea that you are worthless.

> In her relationships with men, Karen became jealous when her boyfriend of the moment talked to other women at social events attended by her friends. While it was the case that Karen saw these women as a threat to her current relationship, she was also preoccupied with, as she put it, her boyfriend 'taking the mickey' in front of her friends. For Karen and other people for whom shame is a component of unhealthy jealousy, not only do they believe that their partner must not show an interest in members of the opposite sex, they also believe that their partners must not be seen to show such interest in front of others.

When shame forms a part of the unhealthy jealousy complex of emotions, it has three components:

1 You believe that, when your partner's behaviour towards a member of the opposite sex constitutes a threat to your relationship and is noticed by others, then others will think that this behaviour makes a fool out of you.
2 You believe that these people must not think poorly of you.

3 You believe that if others do think that you are a fool, then this proves that you are a fool.

Having thus considered the different emotions that form the complex emotional response known as unhealthy jealousy, I will now consider the ways in which people behave and tend to act when they are unhealthily jealous.

How you act (or tend to act) when you are unhealthily jealous

As I discussed in Chapter 1, when you experience an emotion you also experience an urge to act in a variety of ways that are consistent with this emotion. These urges to act are known as action tendencies.

Most of the time you go along with these tendencies in your behaviour, but you can also act against them. Indeed, if you were unable to act against your action tendencies, change wouldn't be possible. In this section, I will discuss the way you act or tend to act when you experience unhealthy jealousy. It is crucial that you understand your unhealthy jealousy-related behaviours, for two reasons. First, you can use your urges to act as reminders that you are experiencing unhealthy jealousy and thence work to identify, challenge and change the irrational beliefs that underpin your unhealthy jealousy. Second, you need to understand the impact of your behaviour on your partner when you are experiencing this destructive emotion. For it is often the way you act towards your partner when you are feeling unhealthy jealousy that is so destructive to your relationship.

So what are the major behaviours and action tendencies associated with unhealthy jealousy?

Constant surveillance

When you are with your partner in a situation where you think that another person may pose a threat to your relationship and you experience unhealthy jealousy, you tend to scan the situation constantly for signs of the threat.

Mary was in the pub with her new boyfriend, Malcolm, and two other couples. Because she was experiencing unhealthy jealousy, she kept watching Malcolm to see if he was looking at other women. She also kept a watchful eye on the other women to see if they were looking at Malcolm. Because of her constant surveillance, Mary was unable to concentrate on her friends' conversation.

People who experience unhealthy jealousy often have a distracted air when they are with their partners in a social situation.

Constant questioning

A very common behavioural manifestation of unhealthy jealousy is constant questioning. Partners of those who are unhealthily jealous often complain that their jealous partners frequently give them the third degree. When you are unhealthily jealous, you may well insist on knowing in minute detail aspects of your partner's experience that impinge on the threat to your relationship that you constantly think exists. If your partner goes to an event on his own, for example, it is likely that you will attempt to find out if other women were there, how old they were, what they looked like, who your partner spoke to, whether he found her attractive and so on. If you are with your partner in a situation when other women are present, your questions are more related to what your partner is thinking, since you have greater access to his behaviour. Thus, you are likely to ask your partner such questions as: 'Do you find that women attractive?'; 'If you weren't with me, which of the women here would you want to go out with?'; 'What are you thinking?'; 'Who are you looking at?'; 'Who are you thinking about?', etc.

Behind this line of questioning is your desperation to assure yourself that no threat exists to your relationship, but your inability to be thus reassured means that you will never receive the assurance that you crave, at least in the long term. As I will discuss in the next section, a key feature of unhealthy jealousy is distrust. You find it difficult, if not impossible, to trust your partner in a situation where there are members of the opposite sex present and you are not with your partner, and because you do not have access to your partner's thoughts you find it difficult to trust that your partner is not being unfaithful to you in his mind when you are with him.

Constant checking

When you are unhealthily jealous, you will also experience a tendency to check constantly on your partner, and when opportunities allow, you will actually carry out such checks.

> Keith experienced unhealthy jealousy in his relationship with his wife Martha. When Martha said that she was meeting her girlfriends for a drink after work, Keith was convinced that she was meeting a man. Consequently, Keith would check on Martha's movements and follow her. Despite the fact that Martha always did what she said she was going to do, this had little or no impact on Keith, who suspected that Martha was too clever to be caught.

In these days of itemised telephone bills, it is easy for people who are unhealthily jealous to check on their partner's phone calls. If they discover unrecognized telephone numbers on these bills, they think nothing of dialling the numbers to discover who their partners have been calling. If they discover that the other person is a woman, they will either try to discover the relationship between this person and their partner or they will interrogate their partner until they discover the truth. Of course, they will not readily accept their partner's reassurance that he is not having a romantic relationship with the other woman until they are faced with the truth. Discovering the innocence of a particular relationship does not assure them that their partner is not having a romantic relationship with another woman, only that they have not yet discovered it.

As with questioning, you desperately hope that your checks will prove that no threat exists to your relationship, but you can't convince yourself that this is so. Thus, like Keith, you think that you are being outwitted by your partner who – you think – is skilled in the art of deception.

Setting traps

When you are unhealthily jealous you will experience the urge to set traps to catch your partner out in his deceit, Mandy, one of my clients, was typical in this respect. Here is an example of one of her traps.

> Before going out, leaving her husband on his own in the house, she would pull out a hair from her head, lick it and place the hair on the telephone. On returning she would check that the hair was still in place. If it was not there, she concluded that this meant that her husband had telephoned his lover. Rather than confront him with her suspicions, she would casually ask him if he had made any telephone calls. If he said that he hadn't, she would convince herself that her suspicions were true. This woman did not, for one minute, consider that after a while the hair would dry and float away on its own.

Placing restrictions on your partner

People who are unhealthily jealous and check on and/or set traps for their partners tend not to view themselves as dominant in these relationships. On the other hand, people who are unhealthily jealous and do consider themselves to be dominant in their relationships are more likely to restrict their partners than check up on them or set traps for them.

The most common form of restriction used by people who are unhealthily jealous is geographical restriction. This means that you forbid your partner to go to certain places. These are normally places where you think that your partner would come into contact with members of the opposite sex and where the purpose of such places is for social intercourse (e.g. clubs, pubs and dance halls). People who have a particular problem with unhealthy jealousy tend to be more general in their restrictions, with some banning their partner from any contact with the opposite sex altogether. Before I began to see him for counselling, Derek banned his wife from answering the front door in case she encountered the postman or the milkman. If your unhealthy jealousy reaches such proportions, you definitely require professional help and I strongly suggest that you tell your GP about the full extent of your unhealthy jealousy problem. As you can imagine, the partners of such individuals are frequently very unhappy with their relationship and often refer to their partners as tyrants.

This is apt because, in addition to being unhealthily jealous, such people are also very possessive. They treat their partners as possessions and hardly consider that they are people in their own right. Largely because of their emotional problems, people who are possessive as well as unhealthily jealous find it difficult to think of the other person, so wrapped up are they in their own problems. They rarely think of the unhappiness of their partners other than when this constitutes a threat to THEM. If their partner says to them that he is unhappy, this is only viewed as further proof that their partner is plotting to leave them and therefore they have even more reason to restrict him.

Another form of restriction practised by those who are unhealthily jealous is what I call behavioural restriction. Here, you restrict or ban your partner from engaging in certain activities. For example, Jack allowed Pam to go to dances with her girlfriends, but he banned her from dancing with any men. This is an example of a behavioural restriction without a geographical restriction.

Common behavioural bans that people who experience unhealthy jealousy place on their partners include not talking to members of the opposite sex, not looking or smiling at members of the opposite sex, and not watching TV programmes and/or videos that the person who is unhealthily jealous considers a threat to the relationship in some way. Thus, one of my clients used to turn off the television whenever there was any kind of sexual contact between the actors, including kissing. When I asked her what she found threatening about such scenes, she said the following.

'I can't bear the thought that Frank [her husband] might watch these scenes and get turned on by them. If this happened it would mean that Frank would rather be with the actress than he would be with me, and that would be the end of the relationship because I must be the only woman in the world that Frank fancies.'

Another form of restriction that people who are unhealthily jealous impose on their partners concerns the clothes that their partners wear. I call this dress restriction. This form of restriction is more frequently imposed by men on their partners than by women on their partners. The type of clothes that men ban their partners from wearing fall into two major categories:

1 Clothes that reveal too much (i.e. in the minds of the men concerned) of their partners' bodies or that highlight certain bodily parts. Thus, men who are unhealthily jealous tend to ban their partners from wearing clothes that reveal their partners' legs, breasts and thighs or that highlight these features (e.g. tight, hugging dresses).

2 Clothes that are (in the minds of the men concerned) likely to give other men the 'wrong impression' of their partners. Some of my female clients who have partners who are unhealthily jealous have told me that their partners won't let them wear clothes that their partners think look 'tarty', like red skirts and blouses and black tights and stockings. One or two of my clients have said that their partners have even forbidden them from wearing any make-up whatsoever. Again, what lies behind these bans is the idea that other men would be attracted to these men's partners and that the partners would respond to any advances made to them by the other men, either in deed or in thought.

Retaliation

Some people who are unhealthily jealous and who are convinced that their partners have been unfaithful to them respond by being unfaithful themselves. Most of the time the person concerned has no actual evidence that their partner has been unfaithful, but they tend to regard their inference that infidelity has taken place as a fact and retaliate in kind.

> One of my male clients, Marcus, believed that his girlfriend had been having an affair with her boss and could cite numerous supporting 'facts'. All of his evidence seemed to me to be very circumstantial (e.g. they exchanged birthday cards and his girlfriend's boss once rang over the weekend on an urgent business matter). Marcus experienced a number of unhealthy negative emotions about his girlfriend's relationship with her

boss. He was unhealthily jealous, unhealthily angry and depressed about this situation, and believed that his girlfriend's 'affair' with her boss humiliated him in the eyes of people who knew him. In response to this complex mixture of disturbed thoughts and feelings, Marcus believed that he had to get his own back on his girlfriend, so he starting having an affair with a woman at his workplace.

Such retaliative measures often serve several purposes. They serve, first, as an eye for an eye act of revenge and, second, as a compensatory strategy. Here, these measures serve in the minds of the persons who are unhealthily jealous to raise their shattered self-esteem. In order to prove to themselves that they are still attractive, they go out and do the very thing that they are convinced that their partner has done to them, i.e. have an affair.

Punishing your partner

People who experience unhealthy jealousy may also seek to punish their partners in some way. This is particularly the case when unhealthy anger is a predominant feature of unhealthy jealousy. Such punishment frequently takes the form of verbal aggression, although physical aggression can also occur.

Harold experienced unhealthy jealousy towards his wife, Maureen, and subjected her to constant questioning every evening on her return from work. If he was not satisfied with her answers, he would scream offensive abuse at her, and would also do this if she wore clothes that he disapproved of in defiance of his ban.

Other people who experience unhealthy jealousy seek to punish their partners in less direct ways. Sulking is a particularly common form of indirect punishment here. People sulk for several different reasons, but punishing the other person without telling them why you are doing so is quite a frequent occurrence.

Whenever Marie caught her husband, Lawrence, watching love scenes on the television she would walk out of the room and not talk to him for days on end. When she did begin to talk to him again she told him that he knew she hated him watching love scenes on television, and that his refusal to go along with this meant he was more interested in other women than he was in her.

Other forms of punishing partners employed by people who are unhealthily jealous are particularly mean-spirited. This usually involves deliberately depriving one's partner of something that would give that person pleasure or joy.

Arthur was married to Samantha, who had a 21-year-old son from a previous marriage. Arthur experienced unhealthy jealousy in his relationship with Samantha and forbade her to speak to any men younger than 50 years of age. One day, Arthur came home early from work and found Samantha on the doorstep talking to a milkman who had called attempting to get the family's milk order. Arthur was furiously jealous about this and decided to teach Samantha a lesson. Later that week, Arthur had promised to take Samantha up north to her son's graduation. However, he told her that because she had violated his trust (by talking to the milkman) he had changed his mind and would not take her. He also informed her that she could not go on her own as she was obviously not to be trusted, and refused to give her any money for the train fare. So Samantha missed a very important landmark in her son's life. This proved the straw that broke the camel's back: Samantha decided as a result of this episode to leave Arthur and institute divorce proceedings against him.

This is quite a typical end to relationships where one person is vindictive as a result of unhealthy jealousy. Sooner or later the partner decides that he or she has taken enough and leaves. Rather than taking responsibility for their vindictiveness and the understandable effects that such behaviour eventually has on their partners, people who are vindictive as a result of their unhealthy jealousy feel aggrieved at being treated badly by their partners and become increasingly entrenched in the view that members of the opposite sex cannot be trusted. Such is the egocentric world of people who are unhealthily jealous.

Punishing your rival

While some people's anger-related unhealthy jealousy is directed at their partner, others' is directed at the person whom they see as posing a particular threat to their relationship (henceforth called the rival). It is important to appreciate that the person you see as your rival may in reality pose no threat at all to your relationship. The point is that you think he does, and it is to your inferences that you respond rather than to objective reality, unless the two coincide.

You are likely to punish your rival in ways that are similar to how you might punish your partner. Thus, you might verbally berate your rival or even physically abuse him. While it is less likely that you will withdraw from your rival in a sulky way, you are quite likely to make him suffer in some way.

For example, Eric was very unhealthily jealous of his wife's relationship with two of the men she worked with. Objectively, there was no relationship between Jan, his wife, and these two men other than friendly collegiality. However, Eric was convinced there was something going on between his partner and one of the men, and Eric's money was on Gerry, the more good-looking of the two.

Eric blamed Gerry for initiating the (fictitious) affair and resolved to make him suffer. He punished Gerry by spiking his drinks at Jan's office party and informing the police (anonymously, of course) that Gerry was driving while under the influence of alcohol. The police arrested and charged Gerry, who lost his licence for six months. As Gerry needed his car for work, he also lost his job, something which gave Eric particular satisfaction. As often occurs when the person who is unhealthily jealous punishes his rival, Gerry never discovered who called the police that night. In his behaviour towards Gerry, Eric was displaying passive-aggressive behaviour. He was being aggressive towards Gerry by getting him into trouble with the police and his employers, but did so in a passive way, meaning that he concealed the fact that he was the author of the aggression. In other instances, however, the person who is unhealthily jealous wants his rival to know that he is the one who is responsible for exacting the punishment.

How you think when you are unhealthily jealous

So far I have discussed two types of thinking that are related to unhealthy jealousy. Earlier in this chapter, I explained that you are unhealthily (and healthily) jealous about instances when you think that you face a threat to your relationship with your partner posed by a third person (at A in the ABC framework). Then I explained that the reason why you feel unhealthily jealous is that you hold a set of irrational beliefs about these threats (at B in the ABC framework). Here, I will discuss the fact that these irrational beliefs not only lead you to experience unhealthy jealous feelings (emotional Cs), but also lead you to think in unconstructive ways. This is how you think once you have begun to feel unhealthily jealous. This type of thinking is basically an elaboration of jealous themes and scenarios and serves to prevent you from standing back and looking objectively at the threats to your relationship that you think you are facing.

Distrust and suspiciousness

When you become unhealthily jealous about a threat to your relationship, you tend to underestimate how trustworthy your partner is and your thoughts become filled with suspicions about what he is doing with other women. This distrust and suspicion is heightened when you are faced with uncertainty and are unable to check on what your partner is doing, and often take the form of scenarios in your head where your partner and your rival are sexually and/or emotionally involved. In this respect, there is some research which suggests that women who are unhealthily jealous are more likely than men to think of scenarios where their partner is emotionally involved with another woman, whereas men are more likely to think of scenarios where their partner is sexually involved with another man.

Glenda was supposed to meet her boyfriend, Nick, at their favourite bar at 8 p.m., but after half an hour Nick hadn't arrived. Glenda rang Nick's flat and was told that he had gone out for the evening, at which point Glenda made herself unhealthily jealous. The longer the evening wore on, the more elaborate the scenario inside Glenda's head became. After three hours, Glenda had developed the idea that Nick was with another woman, having a candlelit dinner and exchanging words of endearment. In reality, it transpired that Nick's car had broken down and he had spent three hours waiting for the breakdown service to arrive.

Thinking that your partner has a negative attitude towards you

Once you feel unhealthily jealous, you tend to think that your partner has a negative attitude towards you. If, when you are unhealthily jealous, you are asked what your partner thinks of you, you will reply that she doesn't care for you, she doesn't love you any more (if she ever did), she doesn't find you attractive or she finds you boring and that is why she is interested in someone else.

Thinking distortedly about your partner's behaviour

When you are unhealthily jealous about what you think your partner is doing with your rival, you tend to think very distortedly about her behaviour. You may think, for example, that she has rejected you, betrayed you or made a fool of you. As we have seen, such inferences may be true, but need to be tested out objectively against the available evidence. However, when you experience unhealthy jealousy, you tend to treat these inferences as being true and you rarely stand back and check them out against reality. Your unhealthy jealousy leads you to think in ways that are consistent with the idea that you are facing a serious threat to your relationship with your partner.

Thinking distortedly about your future relationships

When you experience unhealthy jealousy you tend to make negative predictions about any future relationships that you may have. When Simon became unhealthily jealous of his girlfriend's relationship with her boss, he also became quite depressed because he thought that he would not be able to trust any woman again.

Thinking negatively about your own qualities

When you are feeling unhealthily jealous about your relationship with your partner, you will tend to think negatively about your own personal qualities, particularly with reference to relationships. Thus, you may think that you are not good enough for your partner, that you are unattractive or that you are boring. You will also tend to think that you are inferior to your rival in what you have to offer your partner.

Thinking of members of the opposite sex as rivals

When you feel unhealthily jealous about your partner, you will very frequently tend to view members of the opposite sex as rivals. For example, whenever Julian saw his girlfriend, Hilary, talking to other men at a social gathering, he felt unhealthily jealous about what he saw and tended to view all these men as rivals for his girlfriend's affections.

A core feature of unhealthy jealousy: Cognitive consequences at C become inferences at A

So far, I have explained that when you hold irrational beliefs at B in the ABC part of the framework, you will tend to think negatively at C. These negative thoughts at C are known as cognitive consequences. If you tend to experience unhealthy jealousy frequently in your relationships you will tend to bring your irrational beliefs to situations at A. When you do so, you will also tend to bring your cognitive consequences to the inferences that you make at A. This means that your inferences at A will be highly coloured by these cognitive consequences. This is particularly the case when the situations you face at A are ambiguous.

Thus, if you are prone to unhealthy jealousy and you are faced with events that are potentially threatening to your relationship (e.g. you see your partner talking to a member of the opposite sex or you don't know where your partner is), your inferences will be coloured by most of the thinking tendencies discussed above:

- an attitude of distrust and suspiciousness;
- thinking that your partner has a negative attitude towards you;
- thinking negatively about your partner's behaviour;
- thinking negatively about your own personal qualities;
- thinking of members of the opposite sex as rivals.

It is as if you bring to these events the following rules that have a great influence on the inferences that you make about these events at A:

- My partner cannot be trusted with other men.
- My partner does not find me attractive, lovable and/or interesting and is bound to find other men more attractive, lovable and/or more interesting than me.
- My partner is bound to reject me, betray me or make a fool of me.
- I have far less to offer my partner than other men do.
- All men are predatory and are bound to try to steal my partner away from me.

The presence of these rules, created as they are by your irrational beliefs described earlier (see pp. 19–22), explains why you are so threatened in your relationships if you are prone to unheatlhy jealousy. For if you are so prone, you tend to see threats to your relationship everywhere, even though objectively no such threats exist. In order to overcome unhealthy jealousy, it follows that you have to modify these rules and the irrational beliefs that play such a large part in creating them.

When you are prone (and not prone) to unhealthy jealousy

If you experience unhealthy jealousy, it is important for you to determine how prone you are to this destructive emotion. When you experience unhealthy jealousy infrequently in a small number of specific situations, then you can be said not to be particularly prone to unhealthy jealousy. On the other hand, if you experience unhealthy jealousy frequently in a large number of situations then you can be said to be prone to unhealthy jealousy.

Inferences

If you are not particularly prone to unhealthy jealousy, you tend to experience this form of jealousy only when you have clear evidence that another person poses a threat to your relationship (e.g. when you catch your boyfriend in bed with another woman or you catch your girlfriend having a candlelit dinner with another man when she said she was visiting her mother). However, you do not feel unhealthily jealous when your partner is, for example, talking to other men at social gatherings or even dancing with other men at parties unless there is clear evidence that she is interested in them romantically or sexually. You take at face value the contact that your partner has with members of the opposite sex, and if you do have your suspicions you do not regard them as facts. Rather, you check out your suspicions with your partner and you tend to believe what she says if her explanation accords with the available data.

> For example, one day Ralph, who is not particularly prone to unhealthy jealousy, suddenly encountered his girlfriend in the company of another man at a restaurant. When he asked her later what she was doing, she replied that she was with one of her work clients who wanted to discuss some business arrangements over lunch. Ralph believed her.

However, if Ralph kept encountering his girlfriend with the same man or with different men in unexpected situations he would probably experience unhealthy jealousy, partly because he would begin to think that his relationship was under threat from a third party or parties. Thus, if you are not particularly prone to unhealthy jealousy you tend to give your partner the benefit of the doubt on a number of occasions, but you would not continue to do so indefinitely. After a while you would begin to distrust her.

However, if you are prone to unhealthy jealousy, as discussed earlier, you tend to see threats to your relationship everywhere.

Rules

If you are not particularly prone to unhealthy jealousy, you would not have the same set of rules that people who are prone to unhealthy jealousy have. Rather, you would have the following set of rules.

- My partner can be trusted with other men, although I do not rule out the possibility that she may prove untrustworthy at some point.
- My partner does find me attractive, lovable and/or interesting, but she may find some other men attractive, lovable and/or more interesting than me.
- My partner will probably not reject me, betray me or make a fool of me, but I cannot rule out the possibility that she might one day do so.
- I have at least as much to offer my partner as other men do, and probably a lot more.
- Some men are predatory and are bound to try to steal my partner away from me, but most aren't.

This more flexible set of rules means that you do not see threats to your relationship that are not clearly present. Compare the above rules to those held by people who are prone to experience unhealthy jealousy. I have already outlined these on p. 40, but repeat them here so you can make a direct comparison with the rules held by those who are not particularly prone to unhealthy jealousy. In doing so, you will easily understand why those who are prone to unhealthy jealousy infer threats to their relationship far more readily than those who are not as prone.

- My partner cannot be trusted with other men.
- My partner does not find me attractive, lovable and/or interesting and is bound to find other men more attractive, lovable and/or more interesting than me.
- My partner is bound to reject me, betray me or make a fool of me.

- I have far less to offer my partner than other men do.
- All men are predatory and are bound to try to steal my partner away from me.

Irrational beliefs

When you are not particularly prone to unhealthy jealousy and you actually experience this destructive emotion, you are likely to do so when you encounter a situation where another person actually poses a threat to your relationship with your partner, and you do so because you hold a set of specific irrational beliefs about this specific situation.

However, when you are prone to experience unhealthy jealousy, you have a set of general irrational beliefs about a much broader number of situations than is the case when you are not so prone.

Unhealthy negative emotions

Earlier, I mentioned that from one perspective unhealthy jealousy is a composite emotion comprising anxiety, unhealthy anger, hurt, depression and shame. It follows from this perspective that if you are prone to unhealthy jealousy then you will experience these unhealthy negative emotions more frequently than if you are not particularly prone to unhealthy jealousy. In this latter case, you will still experience these other emotions when you feel unhealthily jealous, but you will do so less frequently and with less intensity than if you are prone to unhealthy jealousy.

Action tendencies and behaviour

On pp. 28–37, I discussed how people tend to act when they experience unhealthy jealousy. In particular, I mentioned the following actions and action tendencies:

- constant surveillance
- constant questioning
- checking
- setting traps
- placing restrictions on your partner
- retaliation

- punishing your partner
- punishing your rival.

If you are not particularly prone to unhealthy jealousy, you will tend to act in these ways when you actually experience unhealthy jealousy, but you will do so only when it is clear that you are actually facing a threat to your relationship posed by a third person. Thus, you will tend to behave in the above-mentioned ways far more frequently when you are prone to unhealthy jealousy, because you think that your relationship is under threat far more frequently than you do if you are not as prone.

In my counselling work with clients who experience unhealthy jealousy I have noted that those who are particularly prone to this destructive emotion act in the above ways far more compulsively than those who are not thus prone.

Thinking consequences of unhealthy jealousy

Earlier I showed that when you experience unhealthy jealousy, you then tend to think in the following ways:

- You tend to be distrustful and suspicious of your partner.
- You tend to think that your partner has a negative attitude towards you.
- You tend to think negatively of your partner's behaviour.
- You tend to think negatively about your future relationships.
- You tend to think negatively about your own qualities.
- You tend to think of members of the opposite sex as rivals.

If you are not particularly prone to unhealthy jealousy, you will tend to think in the above ways when you actually experience unhealthy jealousy, but since you will only experience this form of jealousy when you have clear evidence that another person poses a threat to your relationship with your partner, you will not think in these ways frequently. However, if you are prone to experience unhealthy jealousy, then you will think in these ways much more frequently because you see threats to your relationship around every corner. Also, if you are prone to unhealthy jealousy, your subsequent thinking will be much more unrealistic and more all-encompassing than if you are not thus prone. For example, when you think of members of the opposite sex as rivals, you will think of many more people as threats if you are prone to experience unhealthy jealousy than if you are not thus prone. Also, in the former case, you will tend to see the threats posed by these people as more serious than in the latter case.

In conclusion, the differences between those who are prone to unhealthy jealousy and those who experience this destructive emotion but do so infrequently are as follows:

1 The former perceive threats to their relationship with their partner posed by members of the opposite sex very frequently and often in the absence of any hard evidence, whereas the latter perceive such threats when it is clear that they exist.
2 The former have a set of rules that help to explain why they often perceive threats to their relationship, whereas the latter have a very different, more flexible set of rules which means that they are not prone to see threats to their relationship unless there is clear evidence that such threats exist.
3 The former hold a set of general unhealthy jealousy-related irrational beliefs, which have led to the development of the rules mentioned above and which help to explain why they perceive threats to their relationship so readily, while the latter hold a set of specific irrational beliefs about readily identifiable threats.
4 The former will experience other unhealthy negative emotions like anxiety, unhealthy anger, hurt, depression and shame more frequently and probably with greater intensity than the latter.
5 The two groups act similarly when they feel unhealthily jealous, but the former act in such ways far more frequently, given their greater proneness to perceive threats to their relationship than the latter group. The former also tend to be more compulsive in their unhealthy jealousy-related behaviour than the latter group.
6 The two groups also think similarly once they have begun to feel unhealthily jealous, but once again those who are prone to this destructive emotion do so more frequently than those who are not thus prone. Also, the former group's thinking tends to be more

unrealistic and more all-encompassing than the thinking of the latter group.

This ends my discussion of the ABCs of unhealthy jealousy. In the next chapter, I will consider the nature of what may be called healthy jealousy.

3

The ABCs of Healthy Jealousy

One of the problems with the English language is that it does not have suitable words for a number of healthy negative emotions, i.e. emotions that are negative in tone but represent constructive feeling responses to negative activating events. For example, shame is an unhealthy negative emotion, but we do not have a good word for its healthy negative alternative. Given this, I use the word 'disappointment' to denote this alternative. Similarly, we have to differentiate between unhealthy anger and healthy anger because we do not have an appropriate word to denote a type of anger that is negative in tone, constructive both in nature and in its consequences and that can be intense in the face of very negative activating events.

In this book, I differentiate between unhealthy jealousy and healthy jealousy, because we do not have a good word for an emotion that we experience when we face a threat to our relationship with our partner, as posed by a third person, that is negative in tone and once again constructive in both nature and effects. So, in this book, I am using the term 'healthy jealousy' to denote this emotion. I have already used the term 'unhealthy jealousy' to denote an emotion that we experience when we face (or, more often, think we face) a threat to our relationship with our partner, as posed by a third person, that is negative in tone and destructive in nature and in its effects.

What we feel healthily jealous about

In the previous chapter, I explained that you feel unhealthily jealous about a threat to your relationship with your partner that is posed by another person, usually, but of course not always, a member of the same sex as you. In the ABC framework, this threat is an A (or activating event). Since you feel healthily jealous about exactly the same situation, you cannot distinguish healthy jealousy from unhealthy jealousy (which, you will recall, are Cs in the ABC framework) by looking at what we feel unhealthily and healthily jealous about. In REBT, we say that you cannot understand C just by referring to A.

Having said this, when you feel healthily jealous you are more likely to experience this emotion when you face a threat to your relationship that is real rather than imagined. In this case, people who feel healthily jealous are more similar to those who feel unhealthily jealous but are not particularly prone to experience this destructive emotion, than they are to those who are prone to experience unhealthy jealousy.

What is the nature of the threat in healthy jealousy? Exactly what it is in unhealthy jealousy, again with one important exception: that more often you have definite evidence that the threat exists in healthy jealousy, whereas in unhealthy jealousy, and particularly if you are prone to experience this destructive emotion, the threat exists more in your mind than in reality. So the nature of the threat in healthy jealousy is fourfold.

1 You have definite evidence that another person is about to replace you in the affections of your partner and that your partner will leave you for the other person.
2 You have definite evidence that your partner finds another person more attractive than you, and while you don't think that she will go off with the other person you consider that you will be displaced as the most important person in her life. Here, while you are not threatened by your partner's interest in the other person, you are threatened by the fact that you will no longer be the most important person in her life.
3 It is important to you that your partner is interested only in you and you are threatened by any definite interest that she shows in another person. Here, while exclusivity is important to you, you do not necessarily think that your partner is going to leave you.
4 It is important to you that no-one shows any serious interest in your partner and you are threatened by any serious interest that another person shows in your partner. Here, your focus is on the other person rather than on your partner.

Since healthy jealousy is mainly experienced in relation to actual threats (i.e. threats to your relationship for which you have clear-cut evidence), you are less likely to experience this healthy emotion about future threats than present and past threats, for future threats are by their very nature inferential, for which you have little evidence. If you are prone to unhealthy jealousy, you can and often do experience this unhealthy emotion about possible threats to your relationship posed by people that your partner hasn't even yet met.

Why we feel healthily jealous

I have made the point that people feel healthily jealous most often about an actual threat to an important relationship posed by a third person. Once again, however, I want to stress that what we feel healthily jealous about is not the same issue as why we feel healthily jealous. Let me again use the ABC part of the ABCDEFG framework to explain what I mean.

You will remember that A stands for an activating event (actual or inferred), B stands for your beliefs about this activating event and C stands for the emotional, behavioural and thinking consequences of your beliefs about A. Applying the ABC part of the overall framework, this means that when you experience healthy jealousy (at C) about an actual (or perceived) threat to your relationship (at A) you experience this healthy reaction not because of the threat itself but because of the beliefs that you hold about this threat.

So, A does not determine C on its own. Rather, your beliefs about A largely determine C. As I pointed out in Chapter 2, this does not mean that A is irrelevant. Far from it – if a threat to your relationship did not exist then you wouldn't experience healthy jealousy. What it means is that the existence of a threat to your relationship, on its own, does not account for your experience of healthy jealousy. To experience healthy jealousy you have to hold a set of rational beliefs about that threat.

Let me sum up my position on this point.

1 Facing a threat to your relationship is a necessary condition for

healthy jealousy to be experienced, but it is not sufficient for this emotional state to be experienced.

2 Facing a threat to your relationship plus holding a set of rational beliefs are necessary and sufficient conditions for healthy jealousy to be experienced.

Having argued that the determining factor in healthy jealousy is the set of rational beliefs about the threat that you face to your relationship, let me consider in greater detail the nature of these rational beliefs. You will recall from Chapter 1 that REBT emphasizes four such beliefs: full preferences; anti-awfulizing beliefs; high frustration tolerance (HFT) beliefs; and acceptance beliefs, where the person accepts him or herself, other people and/or life conditions. While these four rational beliefs are interlinked, I will deal with them one at a time. I will begin with full preferences, because Albert Ellis, the founder of Rational Emotive Behaviour Therapy, argues that if rational beliefs are at the heart of psychological health including healthy jealousy, then full preferences are at its very core.

Full preferences

Holding full preferences is at the very core of a variety of healthy negative emotions and this is certainly the case in healthy jealousy. There are two major components of a full preference: an assertion of what you prefer, and an acknowledgment that you do not have to have your preference met. If only the first component is present, then it is entirely possible for you to transform what I call a partial preference into a rigid demand. For example, if you hold the belief: 'I would prefer it if my partner was only interested in me, but there is no reason why she must not be interested in anyone else', this is a full preference because you assert what you want (i.e. 'I would prefer it if my partner was only interested in me') and you acknowledge that you do not have to have your preference met (i.e. 'but there is no reason why she must not be interested in anyone else'). If you only asserted the partial preference (i.e. 'I would prefer it if my partner was only interested in me') then it would be easy for you to transform this partial preference into a rigid demand (e.g. 'I would prefer it if my partner was only interested in me and therefore she must not be interested in anyone else').

Let me now give you several examples of the main full preferences that underpin healthy jealousy.

'I would prefer it if my partner was only interested in me, but there is no reason why she must not be interested in anyone else.'

'My partner is allowed to find other people attractive, and while I want her to find me more attractive than anyone else, this doesn't mean that she must not find someone else more attractive than me.'

'I would much prefer it if I was the only person that my partner has ever been in love with, but this doesn't have to be the case.'

'I would rather know for certain that my partner is not in the company of other men, but I don't need to know this.'

'I would rather know for certain that my partner is not thinking about anyone of the opposite sex, but I don't need such reassurance.'

'I would rather that my partner not engage in activities with members of the opposite sex, and I would prefer it if these activities were exclusive to our relationship, but I don't have to have my preferences met.'

'I would prefer it if no other woman showed interest in my partner, but this does not have to be the case.'

Anti-awfulizing beliefs

Anti-awfulizing beliefs are flexible evaluations of badness which allow for things to be worse. According to Albert Ellis, these beliefs stem from one's full preferences. I will go over the list that I presented when discussing full preferences and show how anti-awfulizing beliefs fit into the picture.

'I would prefer it if my partner was only interested in me, but there is no reason why she must not be interested in anyone else.

51

If she is interested in someone else that would be very unfortunate, but not terrible.'

'My partner is allowed to find other people attractive, and while I want her to find me more attractive than anyone else, this doesn't mean that she must not find someone else more attractive than me. If she does find someone more attractive than me that would be bad, but it wouldn't be awful.'

'I would much prefer it if I was the only person that my partner has ever been in love with, but this doesn't have to be the case. If she has been in love before, that wouldn't be to my liking, but it wouldn't be horrendous.'

'I would rather know for certain that my partner is not in the company of other men, but I don't need to know this. Not knowing is bad, but not horrible.'

'I would rather know for certain that my partner is not thinking about anyone of the opposite sex, but I don't need such reassurance. It is a misfortune if I don't know that my partner isn't thinking about someone else, but it is hardly the end of the world if I don't know.'

'I would rather that my partner not engage in activities with members of the opposite sex, and I would prefer if it these activities were exclusive to our relationship, but I don't have to have my preferences met. If she does engage in these activities with other men, that would be bad, but hardly terrible.'

'I would prefer it if no other woman showed interest in my partner, but this does not have to be the case. If another woman does show interest in my partner, that would be a bad experience, but not awful.'

High frustration tolerance (HFT) beliefs

HFT beliefs indicate that the person holding them believes that he is able to tolerate a particular event and it is worth his while to do so. Again, Ellis argues that HFT beliefs stem from full preferences as shown in the following:

'I would prefer it if my partner was only interested in me, but there is no reason why she must not be interested in anyone else. If she is interested in someone else, that would be difficult to bear, but I could bear it.'

'My partner is allowed to find other people attractive and, while I want her to find me more attractive than anyone else, this doesn't mean that she must not find someone else more attractive than me. If she does find someone more attractive than me, I would just about be able to deal with that, but I could deal with it.'

'I would much prefer it if I was the only person that my partner has ever been in love with, but this doesn't have to be the case. If she has been in love before, I could put up with it, although it would be tough.'

'I would rather know for certain that my partner is not in the company of other men, but I don't need to know this. Not knowing would be hard to put up with, but I could do so.'

'I would rather know for certain that my partner is not thinking about anyone of the opposite sex, but I don't need such reassurance. I could stand not knowing that my partner isn't thinking about someone else, although it would be difficult.'

'I would rather that my partner not engage in activities with members of the opposite sex, and I would prefer it if these activities were exclusive to our relationship, but I don't have to have my preference met. If she does engage in these activities with other men, I could tolerate that with a struggle.'

'I would prefer it if no other woman showed interest in my partner, but this does not have to be the case. If another woman does show interest in my partner, I could bear it, although it would be hard.'

Acceptance beliefs

Acceptance beliefs involve acknowledging that you and other people are too complex to be given a global negative rating, although parts of yourself and others can be rated. Once again, according to Ellis, acceptance beliefs stem from full preferences (as shown below).

'I would prefer it if my partner was only interested in me, but there is no reason why she must not be interested in anyone else. If she is interested in someone else, that would not mean that I am worthless. I can accept myself whether or not she is interested in someone else.'

'My partner is allowed to find other people attractive and, while I want her to find me more attractive than anyone else, this doesn't mean that she must not find someone else more attractive than me. If she does find someone more attractive than me, it doesn't mean that I am less worthy than the other person. We are of equal worth, but unequal in attractiveness in the eyes of one person.'

'I would much prefer it if I was the only person that my partner has ever been in love with, but this doesn't have to be the case. If she has been in love before, this doesn't mean that I am less lovable than the other person. My lovableness is not defined by being the only person that my partner has ever loved.'

'I would rather that my partner not engage in activities with members of the opposite sex, and I would prefer it if these activities were exclusive to our relationship, but I don't have to have my preferences met. If she does engage in these activities with other men, other people may think that I am a fool, but they'd be wrong. I can accept myself as a fallible human being even if other people can't.'

'I would prefer it if no other woman showed interest in my partner, but this does not have to be the case. If another woman does show interest in my partner, she is not a bitch. Rather, she is a fallible human being who is doing something that I disapprove of.'

According to this analysis, then, threats to our relationships (real or inferred) posed by third persons do not, on their own, explain why we feel healthily jealous. Rather, we feel healthily jealous because we hold one or more rational beliefs about such threats.

Healthy jealousy and other healthy negative emotions

Up to now I have again viewed healthy jealousy as an emotion in its own right. Using the ABC part of the ABCDEFG framework I have shown the following:

A = Real (or inferred) threat to your relationship posed by a third person

B = Rational beliefs (full preferences, anti-awfulizing beliefs, HFT beliefs, acceptance beliefs)

C = Healthy jealousy.

As I mentioned in Chapter 2, there is another view in the field of psychology, however, which states that healthy jealousy is not a single emotion. Rather, it is a complex mixture of different emotions. Taking this view again, I will now discuss those healthy negative emotions which make up healthy jealousy. In doing so, I will discuss concern, healthy anger, sorrow, sadness and disappointment, since these seem to be the major emotions that comprise healthy jealousy. As I discuss these healthy emotions, I will return to the examples that I examined on pp. 23–28 and discuss the examples as if the people concerned experienced healthy negative emotions instead of the unhealthy negative emotions they actually experienced.

Concern

If you experience healthy jealousy, the chances are that you will be concerned when an actual threat to your relationship seems likely. Being concerned rather than anxious, you will not be constantly vigilant for signs that your partner may be interested in someone else or that someone else may be interested in your partner, as you would be if you were anxious. In addition, you will not read threat into even the most innocent interchanges between your partner and members of the opposite sex. Being concerned, you will be vigilant when it becomes clear that your partner is interested in someone else or someone is interested in your partner. You will be able to relax when you are with your spouse in mixed company unless a threat to your relationship is clearly on the horizon. You will also be able to relax when you are not in the company of your partner, because you basically trust your partner unless you have good reason not to.

In the case of Marion that I discussed on pp. 23–24, you will recall that as a result of Marion's jealousy she and her husband, Vic, spent little time with other people (because Marion believed that she couldn't bear the thought of Vic looking at and talking to other women) and Vic spent very little time apart from Marion (because Marion believed that she couldn't bear the thought of Vic being in the same room as other women). However, even being together with Vic in their own home did not lessen Marion's anxiety. For example, she was constantly nervous while they were both watching the television in case an attractive female would appear on the TV screen, and she was even anxious while they were both reading separate books in case Vic read a sexy scene in his book and wished that he was with the woman in the novel rather than with Marion. She was anxious when they were doing nothing in case Vic started thinking about an attractive woman, and she was anxious about going to bed in case Vic would dream of another woman. Even when they made love, she couldn't relax because she was scared that Vic was thinking of making love to another woman when he was making love to her.

If Marion experienced healthy jealousy instead of unhealthy jealousy, her life and that of Vic would have been very different. First, they would have been able to spend time with other people; Marion would be able to tolerate the possibility of Vic looking at and talking to other women since these events would not pose threats to her relationship with Vic unless she had clear evidence that she had cause to be concerned. Vic would have been able to spend time apart from Marion because she would not find the thought of him being in the same room as other women threatening. Marion would have been able to relax with Vic in their own home, even when they were both watching the television and an attractive female came on the TV screen, since she would not have immediately jumped to the conclusion that Vic found the woman more attractive than her; even if he did, she would tend to conclude that this would not mean that he would leave her at the first opportunity. In addition, Marion would be at ease when Vic was reading a book even if he read a sex scene, since again she would not conclude that he would rather be with the woman in the novel than with her. If Marion was healthily jealous, she would be able to relax when they made love, because she would not be focused on the idea that Vic was thinking of making love to another woman when he was making love to her.

This revised scenario shows quite clearly that when you are healthily jealous, you will be concerned about the possibility of the existence of a threat to your relationship, but anxiety will not be your constant companion. The feelings of concern that form part of the healthy jealousy complex of emotions have three major components:

1 A real threat to what is important to you.
2 A preference that the threat does not exist, but no dogmatic insistence that it must not exist.
3 The idea that it would be bad, but not terrible, if the threat materialized.

The latter two components mean that you would perceive a threat to your relationship only when it clearly exists.

Healthy anger

Healthy anger is another emotion that forms a part of healthy jealousy. In Chapter 2, I argued that healthy anger involves you attempting to deal with situations you don't like in ways that demonstrate your respect for the other person, whereas unhealthy anger involves you imposing your will in ways that condemn the other person.

While people who frequently experience unhealthy jealousy often have rules that other people, in particular their partners, have to live by, if you experience healthy jealousy your rules are much more flexible. While you probably do have a set of preferences for how you want your partner and other people to behave, you do not demand that they have to behave in these ways.

You will recall that on pp. 24–25 I discussed Bernadette and Paul's situation. They would sometimes go down to their local for a few drinks and Bernadette, who had a long-standing problem with unhealthy jealousy, had a rule that it was wrong for Paul to look at other women in the pub when he was with her. Bernadette would make herself unhealthily angry by her insistence that Paul had to abide by this rule, and when she thought that he had violated the rule she would subject him to a tirade of verbal abuse mixed with accusations thinly disguised as questions.

'How dare you ogle that woman when you know I don't like it? I told you last time we were out that I find it offensive. Why are you doing this to me? You really are a bastard, Paul. I know you'd rather be with her than me. But why do you have to make it so obvious?'

But let's imagine that Bernadette experienced healthy anger rather than its unhealthy form. What would have been the difference? She would still prefer it if Paul did not look at other women when they were out at the pub, but she would not demand that he must not do so. Since her belief about Paul's behaviour was flexible and not rigid, she would not pay that much attention when he glanced at other women, but she would draw the line when it was clear that he was ogling them.

If he did ogle other women she would healthily confront him as follows:

'Paul, I would much prefer it if you did not ogle women when we are out together. What you do when you are on your own is your affair, but please can we agree that while you are out with me you don't do that?'

Note the difference between what Bernadette said here and what she actually said when she was unhealthily angry. When she was healthily angry, Bernadette restricted her comments to the situation and did not make any inferences about Paul preferring to be with other women. She indicated that she didn't like Paul's behaviour and requested that he change it. Note also that she did not condemn Paul as a person. However, when Bernadette was unhealthily angry, she did infer that Paul preferred to be with another woman. Indeed, she assumed that this was a fact, rather than a hypothesis to be tested out. Furthermore, she did condemn Paul and didn't request but demanded a change in his behaviour.

The healthy anger that forms a part of the healthy jealousy complex of emotions has three major components:

1 A rule of conduct for the partner to follow. This rule either prescribes behaviour (i.e. indicates the behaviour the partner is expected to follow) or prohibits behaviour (i.e. indicates the behaviour that the partner is expected to refrain from). This rule is usually far less prescriptive and prohibitive than that found in unhealthy jealousy.
2 A preference that your partner abides by this rule, but an acknowledgment that he doesn't have to do so.
3 The expression of an assertive, non-condemnatory attitude when the partner breaks the rule.

Sorrow

When sorrow is a feature of healthy jealousy, you think that your partner has betrayed you and you consider that you have done nothing to deserve this unfair treatment, but you hold a set of rational beliefs about your undeserved fate.

Let me reconsider the case of Peter and imagine that he felt sorrowful rather than hurt. If you recall (see pp. 25–26) I discussed that as soon as Peter and June got married, Peter began to show signs of unhealthy jealousy. Peter was unemployed while June had a well-paid professional job, a situation which fuelled Peter's insecurity and his unhealthy jealousy. Because he had a lot of time on his hands, Peter spent long periods of time on his own thinking of all the men at her work that June was flirting with. When June came home, Peter interrogated her concerning what she did that day and who she spoke to. After a while, June refused to give

Peter a blow-by-blow account of her interactions, a situation to which Peter responded with anger and then hurt. Peter felt hurt because he considered June's refusal to tell him about her day as an undeserved betrayal of trust. When this happened, Peter became sullen and would not talk to June for hours.

If Peter felt sorrowful instead of hurt, he would still ask June to tell him about her day, but would not ask her for a blow-by-blow account of her experiences. He still might consider June's refusal to tell him about her day as an undeserved betrayal of trust, but he would feel sorrowful rather than hurt about this. Consequently, rather than becoming sullen and sulky, Peter would tell June that as he was alone all day, in his opinion it was unfair of her to refuse to tell him about her day. Thus, he would express his feelings rather than shutting down the channel of communication between them.

The feelings of sorrow that form a part of the healthy jealousy complex of emotions have three major components:

1 The idea that your partner has betrayed you and that you do not deserve this treatment.
2 A preference that she does not do this, together with an acknowledgment that she has the right to act in this unfair manner.
3 A recognition that you are in a poor situation without an accompanying 'poor me' attitude.

Sadness

When sadness is a feature of healthy jealousy, you tend to focus on the idea that while your partner may want to go off with someone else, this would be a sad loss, but you could accept yourself as a fallible human being rather than an unlovable, worthless person if this were to happen. In addition, you do not assume that you will always have difficult relationships with the opposite sex.

The feelings of sadness that form a part of the healthy jealousy complex of emotions have three major components:

1 The inference that you may lose your partner to someone else.
2 The belief that you do not want this to happen, but you do not demand that this must not happen.

3 The belief that you are still a fallible human being if you lose your partner to someone else, which you do not regard as inevitable. If it does happen, you do not assume that you will inevitably lose any partners that you may have in the future.

Disappointment

When disappointment is a feature of healthy jealousy, you are concerned, but not overly so, about how others might view you if you lost your partner. If you did lose your partner to someone else you could accept yourself and would not view yourself as a diminished, defective or disgraced person.

If you recall, on p. 27 I discussed the case of Karen who became unhealthily jealous when her boyfriend of the moment talked to other women at social events attended by her friends. While it was the case that Karen saw these women as a threat to her current relationships, she was also preoccupied with, as she put it, her boyfriend 'taking the mickey' in front of her friends. Karen not only believed that her partner must not show an interest in members of the opposite sex, she also believed that her partner must not be seen to show such interest in front of others. If he did, she thought that this would reveal her as a fool in front of her friends.

If Karen felt disappointment rather than shame, she would still not like it when her boyfriend of the moment talked to other women at social events attended by her friends, but would not think that he was 'taking the mickey' in front of her friends. She would have preferred it if her boyfriend didn't do this, but wouldn't insist that he mustn't do so. If he did so, she would not consider that this revealed her as a fool in front of others. Rather, she would accept herself even if her friends thought she was being made a fool of.

When disappointment forms a part of the healthy jealousy complex of emotions, it has three components:

1 You have clear evidence that your partner's behaviour towards a member of the opposite sex constitutes a threat to your relationship, and you think that this will be noticed by others who may think that this behaviour makes a fool out of you.

2 If it becomes clear that others do think poorly of you for losing your partner to another person, you prefer them not to think of you in this way, but you do not demand that they must not do so.
3 You do not believe that you are a fool even if others think of you in this way. Rather, you accept yourself in the face of others' negative attitude towards you when this is the case.

Having thus considered the different emotions that form the complex emotional response known as healthy jealousy, I will now continue by considering the ways in which people behave and tend to act when they are healthily jealous.

How you act (or tend to act) when you are healthily jealous

In the previous chapter, I considered how you act or tend to act when you are unhealthily jealous. In particular, I discussed the following unhealthily jealous-related actions and action tendencies:

- constant surveillance
- constant questioning
- checking
- setting traps
- placing restrictions on your partner
- retaliation
- punishing your partner
- punishing your rival.

I argued in that chapter that the main reason you tend to act in these destructive ways when you are unhealthily jealous is because you hold a set of irrational beliefs about the threat that you actually face (or think you face) to your relationship with your partner. So far, in the present chapter, I have discussed healthy jealousy which, as you have seen, stems from a set of rational beliefs about this threat. If destructive behaviour stems from irrational thinking in unhealthy jealousy, we should find an altogether more constructive set of actions and action tendencies in healthy jealousy and by and large this is the case.

Testing out your inferences

When you are unhealthily jealous (and particularly if you are prone to unhealthy jealousy) you tend to think that your relationship is, in reality, under threat precisely because you think that it is. You will recall that, in Chapter 1, I argued that frequently we form inferences about reality at point A in the ABCDEFG framework, and ideally we need to treat these inferences as hunches about reality that need to be tested rather than as incontrovertible facts. Thus, when you are unhealthily jealous you regard your inferences as facts and proceed to act accordingly.

However, when you are healthily jealous you are much more likely to regard your inferences as hunches rather than as facts, and you will proceed to test these out with your partner, even if you are quite sure that your relationship is under threat. In checking or testing out your inferences with your partner, you will tend to spell out the evidence that you have in support of the idea that your relationship with your partner is under threat. The evidence that you provide will tend to relate to objective events that most people would agree would constitute a threat to your relationship, and you will tend to describe this evidence in a non-accusatory manner.

This compares with how you tend to behave when you are unhealthily jealous. Here, you tend to accuse your partner of things that most people would not think of as constituting clear evidence of a threat to your relationship (e.g. 'You looked at that woman'). Also, what you accuse your partner of involves your subjective inference of his objective behaviour and often involves mind-reading (e.g. 'I could tell by the way that you looked at that woman that you fancy her more than you fancy me and that you would rather be with her').

Jenny saw her husband, Bill, dancing very closely with another woman at her firm's annual dance. She knew that this other woman had a reputation for trying to seduce other women's husbands and she also knew that her husband had had a bit too much to drink that evening. She felt healthily jealous about the event and about any future contact that Bill might have with her work colleague.

The next day, Jenny checked out with Bill her inference that he fancied the other woman. He said quite firmly that he didn't, but agreed that he had had too much to drink the night before and apologised for his behaviour. Two days later, he told Jenny that her work colleague had called round when she was on a late shift at work and he had told the woman that he wasn't interested in her, an account which Jenny accepted and she soon forgot about the incident.

Had Jenny experienced unhealthy jealousy about the incident at her firm's dance, she would have been more likely to accept as a fact her inference that Bill fancied the other woman and would have tended to view all subsequent events as confirming this 'fact'. Instead, because she experienced healthy jealousy as opposed to unhealthy jealousy she was able to treat her inference as a hypothesis about reality rather than as an indisputable fact.

Assertion

We have already seen that unhealthy anger can be a central component of unhealthy jealousy (see pp. 24–25), whereas when you experience healthy jealousy you are more likely to feel healthily angry (see pp. 57–59). This healthy anger allows you to be assertive with your partner concerning events or issues about which you are displeased. When you assert yourself with your partner you tell her how you feel about something that involves her in a way that is non-accusatory, shows respect for her and, most importantly, does not hold her responsible for your feelings. You also request rather than demand a change in the other person's behaviour.

Benjamin was concerned about the amount of time that his girlfriend, Jane, was spending with Roland, one of her male friends. Although he accepted her assurance that she wasn't interested in him, romantically or sexually, he had heard on the grapevine that her male friend did of late have growing romantic feelings towards her. Benjamin felt healthy jealousy about this threat to his relationship with Jane and this enabled him to assert himself with her as follows:

'Jane, I feel quite concerned about the amount of time you are spending with Roland. I know that you don't fancy him, but I think that he fancies you and is going to try to win you away from me. I feel jealous about the time that you spend with him and would ask you to limit the amount of contact that you have with him.'

Jane replied that Benjamin had no cause for concern, but agreed to limit her contact with Roland in the future. Because of the mature way in which both people handled this threat, this episode served to strengthen their relationship. When Benjamin discovered later that Roland wasn't romantically interested in Jane, he believed this and was quite happy for them both to spend more time with one another.

Since assertion is based on healthy anger, when you are healthily jealous you are unlikely to retaliate against your partner or punish your partner and/or your rival. These three actions and action tendencies stem from unhealthy anger which, as we have seen, is frequently a feature of unhealthy jealousy.

Focused surveillance

When you are healthily jealous about a threat to your relationship, you may well have good evidence that such a threat exists. However, even if you are healthily jealous about a threat that you think exists but for which you do not have objective evidence, the behavioural consequences are the same. Thus you will be on the alert for signs of the existence of this threat, but only in the specific area in which you think your relationship is threatened. In other words, your surveillance is focused on the specific threat that you have (or think you have) located. This compares with the constant surveillance that you carry out when you feel unhealthily jealous, and particularly when you are prone to this destructive emotion.

Hilary thought that her husband, Maurice, was interested romantically in one of her girlfriends, Lorraine, and felt healthily jealous about this. Whenever Hilary and Maurice met with Lorraine at a social gathering, Hilary kept a wary eye open to see whether or not Maurice was talking to Lorraine, and if so, what kind of interaction they were having with one another. However, Hilary was able to give her attention to other friends and was not constantly surveying the situation and scrutinizing Maurice's and Lorraine's whereabouts, as she would have done if she felt unhealthily jealous about the threat posed by Lorraine to her relationship. She also did not generalize this surveillance to other situations, as she would have done if she was particularly prone to unhealthy jealousy.

Focused questioning

In Chapter 2, I showed that when you feel unhealthily jealous about a threat posed to your relationship with your partner, you tend to bombard your partner with a series of questions about her part in this situation. The more you are prone to unhealthy jealousy, the more you will constantly ask your partner about her feelings, thoughts and behaviour concerning your rival. If you are highly prone to unhealthy jealousy, you think you have many such rivals and therefore you will tend to question your partner continually about her feelings, thoughts and behaviour with respect to these rivals. However, if you are healthily jealous you tend to be sparing with your questions and focus them on episodes that you can objectively document.

Focused checking

When you experience healthy jealousy, you tend to have clear-cut evidence that a threat to your relationship actually exists. In this case you may well check on your partner's whereabouts to determine whether or not the threat to your relationship has materialized.

However, you will only check on your partner when you actually have good cause to do so.

Karen heard from her best friend that her partner, Melvin, was seen out with an attractive woman at a restaurant. When she asked Melvin about this, he admitted that he had taken his secretary out for a meal as a thank you for all the overtime that she did for him. Karen felt healthily jealous about this event, but this did not mean that she checked on his whereabouts every time he told her that he was working late at the office, something that she would have done if she had felt unhealthily jealous about Melvin's relationship with his secretary and particularly so if she was highly prone to experiencing this destructive emotion. However, one night Melvin said that he would be home by 10 p.m. after a works 'do', but he hadn't returned by 11.30 p.m. Karen reacted by telephoning the restaurant that her husband and his colleagues had dined at and was told that they had all left at 9.30 p.m. So Karen telephoned her husband's secretary because she thought he may have gone home with her. However, when another man answered, Karen hung up, and a few minutes later Melvin returned home with two of his male work colleagues, slightly inebriated. You can see from this example that Karen's checking behaviour, fuelled as it was by her healthy jealousy, was limited to a specific situation. If she had been unhealthily jealous of her husband's relationship with his secretary, she would have initiated checks much more frequently, particularly if she had been highly prone to unhealthy jealousy.

Other functional behaviours

In Chapter 2, I showed that when you are feeling unhealthily jealous, in addition to constantly questioning, checking on your partner and surveying his whereabouts, you also tend to set traps for him and place restrictions on his behaviour and/or movements. You may well do these things when you are healthily jealous, but only when you have objective evidence that he is very probably involved with someone else and when the other constructive behaviours you have initiated have not allayed your healthy concern. In addition, when you are healthily jealous you are very loath to set traps for your partner or to restrict him, whereas when you are unhealthily jealous – and particularly if you are highly prone to this destructive emotion – you are quite prepared to set traps and restrict him and do so much sooner than you would if you experienced healthy jealousy.

> Tim was healthily jealous about his girlfriend's relationship with her driving instructor. When an anonymous 'well-wisher' rang him to tell him that Mary was having an affair with her instructor, he dismissed it as the 'ravings of a warped mind'. However, when two of his friends told him that they saw Mary kissing someone in a blue car (the same colour as the one owned by the driving instructor), Tim became healthily jealous. This led him to assert himself with Mary and he told her about the anonymous phone call and what his friends had seen. Mary denied that she was having an affair with the other man, and Tim was largely reassured until he began to get a number of telephone calls where the other person replaced the receiver on hearing his voice. Tim's concern deepened and he decided, very reluctantly and as a last resort, to lay a trap for Mary. He told her that he was going away for a few days on business and arranged to phone her at set times. While he was away, Tim engaged the services of a private investigator to check on Mary and video any suspicious encounters that she had. Sure enough, secure in the knowledge that Tim was away, Mary invited the driving instructor to stay the night and the investigator took a video of his arrival at 8.30 p.m. (30 minutes after Tim's planned call to Mary) and his departure at 6.00 the next morning. On seeing the evidence, Tim confronted Mary with it and ended the relationship.

This episode shows clearly that when you are healthily jealous, you are prepared to go to extreme lengths to discover the truth about a possible threat to your relationship, but you will only do so when you have sufficient evidence to support your suspicions and after you have used less extreme methods to discover the truth. This debunks the criticism held by some that healthy jealousy means that you turn a blind eye to possible threats to your relationship. When you are unhealthily jealous, and especially when you are prone to this emotion, you tend to take extreme measures quite willingly, often in the absence of hard evidence that your relationship is threatened by another person.

How you think when you feel healthily jealous

Focused distrust and suspiciousness

You will recall, from Chapter 1, that when you think rationally (at B) about a threat to your relationship (at A) you tend to think realistically at C. As we have seen, when you experience healthy jealousy you do so largely when you have clear-cut evidence that another person poses a threat to your relationship with your partner. Under these conditions you may be distrustful and suspicious of your partner, but only in relation to the person who clearly poses such a threat. In other words, your distrust and suspiciousness are localized, rather than generalized to your partner's relationships with many members of the opposite sex; the latter would be the case if you experienced unhealthy jealousy, and particularly if you are highly prone to do so.

Thinking realistically about your partner's attitude towards you

When you feel healthy jealousy about a threat to your relationship, you will not necessarily conclude that your partner's interest in another person means that she has a negative attitude towards you. Thus, you may think that your partner cares for you, but also cares for the other person. Or you may think that your partner is still interested in you, but also interested in someone else. This is in direct contrast to your thinking in such cases when you experience unhealthy jealousy, where you frequently think that your partner has a negative attitude towards you and cannot comprehend that she can care for or be interested in two people at the same time.

Thinking realistically about your partner's behaviour

If it becomes clear that you have a rival for your partner's affections, when you are healthily jealous about this, you tend to think realistically about your partner's behaviour. You may think, for example, that she has rejected you, betrayed you or made a fool of you (which you would definitely think if you were unhealthily

69

jealous), but you may also conclude other things as well. Thus, you may think that she is going through a difficult time and having difficulty coping with her own feelings. The point is that you will test out your inferences against the available evidence and are able to do this because you are not disturbing yourself unduly about her behaviour.

Thinking realistically about your future relationships

When you experience healthy jealousy, you tend to make realistic predictions about any relationships that you may have in the future. Thus, you may think that if you lose your present partner, you may lose others, but you will also tend to consider that you will be able to make relationships with people who will remain faithful or who will not inevitably leave you for another person.

Thinking realistically about your own qualities

When you are feeling healthily jealous about a threat to your relationship with your partner, you will tend to think realistically about your own personal qualities, particularly with reference to relationships. In contrast to unhealthy jalousy, where you tend to think that you are not good enough for your partner, that you are unattractive and boring or that you have little to offer other women, when you are healthily jealous you still think that you have the same qualities that you had when your partner was involved only with you. You may accept the possibility that your partner no longer has a good opinion of your positive qualities, but you do not conclude that you have lost these qualities as a result. You also accept that your partner may be interested in someone else because you have some unappealing qualities, in which case you are mature enough to acknowledge this possibility and to resolve to deal with these issues.

Thinking realistically about members of the opposite sex as rivals

When you are healthily jealous about your partner, you do not in general view members of the opposite sex as rivals. You may think of a particular person as a rival when you have clear-cut evidence that this is the case, but you do not generalize this to other members of the opposite sex.

Other features of healthy jealousy

In Chapter 2, I explained that it is a core feature of unhealthy jealousy that your cognitive consequences (at C in the ABCDEFG framework) of this destructive emotion become your inferences at A. Thus, when you are unhealthily jealous (and particularly if you are highly prone to this type of jealousy) you tend to bring your distrust and suspiciousness, for example, to events which are ambiguous. Thus, if you see your partner talking to an attractive member of the opposite sex, you will tend to be suspicious of them both and overestimate the degree of threat that exists to your relationship.

When you are healthily jealous, your cognitive consequences of this functional emotion also tend to become your inferences at A. This is why you are able to view ambiguous events in a far more trusting and non-threatening light when you are healthily jealous, and why you only see others posing a threat to your relationship with your partner when there is a clear-cut evidence that such a threat exists.

It is as if you bring to these events the following rules that have a great influence on the inferences that you make about these events at A:

- My partner can basically be trusted with other men unless I have clear-cut evidence to the contrary.
- My partner finds me attractive, lovable and/or interesting and if she finds other men attractive and interesting, she will still find me more attractive and interesting than the other person unless I have clear-cut evidence to the contrary.
- My partner will not reject me, betray me or make a fool of me unless I have clear-cut evidence that this is very likely to happen.
- I have at least as much and probably more to offer my partner than other men do.
- Some men (but by no means all) are predatory and some may try to steal my partner away from me.

As you will note, these rules are very similar to the rules that people who are not highly prone to unhealthy jealousy have (as discussed in Chapter 2). This means that, while it is important to overcome specific instances of unhealthy jealousy even if you are not prone to this destructive emotion, if you are highly prone to unhealthy jealousy it is crucial that you learn to become far less prone to the green-eyed monster. I will discuss how to become less prone to unhealthy jealousy in Chapter 5, but first, in the following chapter, I will suggest ways that you can deal with specific episodes of unhealthy jealousy.

4

How to Deal with Specific Episodes of Unhealthy Jealousy

Whether you are prone to unhealthy jealousy or you experience this destructive emotion only when it is clear that you are facing a threat to your relationship with your partner posed by another person, it is important that you begin the change process by dealing with specific episodes of unhealthy jealousy. This is the focus of this present chapter. In the following chapter I will show how you can become less prone to unhealthy jealousy if you experience this emotion frequently in your life.

What follows is a 13-step guide to overcoming situationally-based unhealthy jealousy. In taking you through these steps I will use the experience of Darren, who selected a specific example of unhealthy jealousy for consideration.

Step 1 Acknowledge that you felt unhealthy jealousy in the situation to be analysed and that this emotion is unhealthy

While this step may seem obvious, in fact it is not; for you may select a situation in which you experienced healthy jealousy rather than unhealthy jealousy. How do you know if your feelings of jealousy are unhealthy? There are three ways of differentiating these two types of jealousy.

First, you need to identify which other emotions comprised your experience of jealousy. As I discussed in Chapters 2 and 3, if you experience unhealthy jealousy, you are likely to experience one or more of the following accompanying unhealthy emotions: anxiety, depression, unhealthy anger, hurt and shame. However, if your feelings of jealousy are healthy, you are likely to experience one or more of the following healthy emotions: concern, sadness, healthy anger, sorrow and disappointment.

Second, you need to identify how you acted (or 'felt' like acting) as a result of your feelings of jealousy. If your jealousy was unhealthy, you acted (or 'felt' like acting) in one or more of the following ways:

- It led you to undertake constant surveillance of your partner.
- It led you to question your partner constantly.
- It led you to check on your partner constantly.
- It led you to set traps for your partner.
- It led you to place restrictions on your partner.
- It led you to retaliate against your partner.
- It led you to punish your partner.
- It led you to punish your rival.

However, if your jealousy was healthy, you acted (or 'felt' like acting) in one or more of the following ways:

- It led you to test out your inferences.
- It led you to assert yourself with your partner.
- If you undertook to carry out surveillance of your partner, your jealousy led you to do so in a focused way and not constantly.
- If you questioned your partner, your jealousy led you to do so in a focused way and not constantly.
- It did not lead you to set traps for your partner unless as a last resort.
- It did not lead you to place restrictions on your partner unless as a last resort.
- It did not lead you to retaliate against your partner.
- It did not lead you to punish your rival.

Third, you need to identify how your jealousy led you to think subsequently. If your jealousy was unhealthy, your subsequent thinking was along one or more of the following lines:

- Your jealousy led you to be generally distrustful and suspicious of your partner.
- It led you to think that your partner had a negative attitude towards you.
- It led you to think in distorted ways about your partner's behaviour.

74

- It led you to think in distorted ways about your future relationships.
- It led you to think negatively about your own qualities.
- It led you to think of members of the opposite sex as rivals.

However, if your jealousy was healthy, your subsequent thinking was along one or more of the following lines:

- If your jealousy led you to be distrustful and suspicious of your partner, this was focused rather than generalized.
- It led you to think realistically about your partner's behaviour.
- It led you to think realistically about your future relationships.
- It led you to think realistically about your own qualities.
- It led you to think realistically about members of the opposite sex as potential rivals.

Darren judged his jealousy to be unhealthy because he 'felt like' placing his girlfriend under constant surveillance and he did, in fact, question her in an obsessive manner. He also thought negatively about his own qualities and tended to see a lot of men as potential rivals. Finally, he retaliated against his partner.

Step 2 Choose a specific example of your unhealthy jealousy and be as concrete as possible

Once you have acknowledged that your jealousy is unhealthy, the next step is for you to select a specific example of this type of unhealthy jealousy. It is very easy for you to think of your unhealthy jealousy in vague terms, but doing so will not help you to identify the specific irrational beliefs that underpin this destructive emotion. Choosing a specific example of your unhealthy jealousy, and being as concrete as possible about it, will enable you to identify your specific irrational beliefs.

Darren chose the following example of his unhealthy jealousy for consideration:
'I went to a party with Kath, my girlfriend, and we were having a good time. Then I went to talk to some friends and when

I went back to find Kath she was laughing and joking with another man. I felt really jealous when I saw them together so I started flirting with another woman to get back at Kath.'

Step 3 Acknowledge that healthy jealousy is the healthy alternative to unhealthy jealousy

In Chapter 1, I discussed the full ABCDEFG model of human disturbance and health. If you recall, G stands for goals that are healthy, realistic and that you wish to strive for. These goals are the healthy alternatives to the unhealthy emotions, behaviours and thoughts that you experience at C in the framework. In this case, it is important that you acknowledge first that there is a healthy alternative to unhealthy jealousy, and second that this alternative is healthy jealousy. If you are facing a threat to your relationship, it is unhealthy for you to feel calm and indifferent about it. If you did, you would have to believe that it doesn't matter to you if you are at risk of losing your relationship with your partner; this would obviously be a lie. If you are unclear that healthy jealousy is the healthy alternative to unhealthy jealousy then I suggest that you re-read Chapter 3.

> Darren acknowledged that the type of jealous reaction he had when he saw Kath laughing and joking with the other man at the party was unhealthy, and understood that a healthier and more realistic reaction would be healthy jealousy where he would not act in a retaliative manner, but would tell Kath how he felt about her behaviour.

Step 4 Accept yourself for feeling unhealthily jealous

Before you start to analyse the concrete example that you have selected, it is important that you ask yourself the following question: Do you depreciate yourself in any way for experiencing unhealthy jealousy? If so, it is important that you deal with this issue before proceeding further with the example of unhealthy jealousy that you have selected. If you bypass your feelings of self-depreciation about experiencing unhealthy jealousy, these feelings will interfere with you working to overcome your jealousy problem.

76

What do you need to do if you are depreciating yourself for feeling unhealthily jealous? First, it is important that you acknowledge that while unhealthy jealousy is a destructive negative emotion, it is a very common one and it is experienced by many people. This means that you are not abnormal for experiencing unhealthy jealousy. Rather, you are a fallible human being for experiencing this emotion, even though it is unhealthy. Second, even if you think of your unhealthy jealousy as a weakness or a sign of immaturity, this does not mean that you are a weak or immature person. Your feelings of unhealthy jealousy are only a part of you and cannot define you. In truth, you are a complex, imperfect person with a jealousy problem and it is important that you remind yourself of this as you work on overcoming this problem. Third, when you depreciate yourself for feeling unhealthily jealous, you are insisting that you must not feel this way in the first place. However, the reality is that you did experience unhealthy jealousy. If there was a law of the universe to prevent you from feeling unhealthily jealous then you would not have experienced this feeling, nor could you have. Obviously, as you did feel unhealthily jealous there is no such law. Remind yourself of this the next time you catch yourself depreciating yourself for feeling unhealthy jealousy.

> Darren realized that he felt ashamed for feeling unhealthily jealous when he saw Kath laughing and joking with the man at the party, and particularly for retaliating in the way that he did. However, he then put into practice the points that I have just made and accepted himself as a fallible human being for feeling and acting as he did, although he recognized that he did not like the way that he felt and particularly disliked his retaliative behaviour. He acknowledged that while he would have preferred to have reacted in a more constructive way, he was neither immune from feeling unhealthy jealousy nor immune from acting in a way that was consistent with these feelings.

Accepting yourself for feeling unhealthy jealousy when you do so will help you to address the issues that led you to feel this way in the first place, so that you can work to experience healthy jealousy instead.

Step 5 Identify the threat to your relationship that you felt most unhealthily jealous about and assume temporarily that this threat is real

You are now ready to identify what you felt most unhealthy jealous about in the specific episode under consideration. From what I have already written, you will know that you are unhealthily jealous about a threat to your relationship with your partner that is posed by another person. Since I am concentrating on romantic jealousy in this book, the other person will be a member of the same sex as you, and this will be true whether you are heterosexual or gay. An exception to this principle will be when your partner is bisexual. Thus, Bill was jealous when Jill, his bisexual partner, began flirting with another woman. However, in this book I will focus on the threat to your relationship posed by a member of your own sex.

Now, if you recall from Chapter 2, I argued that the following different types of threat exist to your relationship:

1 You regard the other person as someone who will replace you in the affections of your partner and think that your partner will leave you for the other person. I will call this threat: LOSING THE RELATIONSHIP.

2 You think that your partner finds the other person more attractive than you and, while you don't think that she will go off with the other person, you consider that you will be displaced as the most important person in her life. Here, while you are not threatened by your partner's interest in the other person, you are threatened by the fact (in your mind) that you will no longer be the most important person in her life. I will call this threat: BEING DEMOTED FROM BEING NUMBER 1.

3 It is important to you that your partner is only interested in you, and you are threatened by any interest that she shows in another person. Here, while exclusivity is important to you, you do not necessarily think that your partner is going to leave you. I will call this threat: LOSING EXCLUSIVITY.

4 It is important that no-one shows any interest in your partner, and you are threatened by any interest that another person shows in her. Here, your focus is on the other person rather than on your

partner. I will call this threat: LOSING THE PLASTIC BUBBLE because the idea that you are the only person in the world who is allowed to be interested in your partner conjures up the notion of you placing your partner in a plastic bubble, safe from the interest of members of your own sex. It is this threat that is often present when possessiveness is a central aspect of unhealthy jealousy.

You will find it helpful to keep these different threats in mind when you strive to identify the aspect of the specific situation under investigation that you were most unhealthily jealous about. When you have found it you have discovered what is known as the critical A. Identifying the critical A is important if you are to get the most out of the steps that follow.

> On reflection, Darren thought he was more jealous about the prospect of losing his exclusive relationship with Kath rather than losing the relationship altogether. This, then, was his critical A.

After you have identified your critical A, it is very important for you to treat it as though it were true, at least for the time being. The reason that it is important you make this assumption is that doing so allows you to identify the irrational beliefs that are at the core of your feelings of unhealthy jealousy. If Darren reassesses his critical A at this point and concludes that Kath's behaviour did not, after all, constitute a threat to the exclusive nature of his relationship with her, then he will stop being unhealthily jealous, but he would not have done so by identifying, challenging and changing his unhealthy jealousy-creating irrational beliefs – which we, in REBT, argue is the better, longer-term solution to his specific unhealthy jealousy problem. If Darren stops feeling unhealthily jealous by concluding that the threat to the exlusive nature of his relationship with Kath was in fact not a threat, for example, he will tend to feel unhealthily jealous if he later reverts to thinking that what happened at the party did constitute such a threat.

So, to reiterate, at this point resist any temptation you may experience to reinterpret your critical A. There will be a better opportunity for you to do so later, after you have modified the irrational beliefs that are at the core of your feelings of unhealthy jealousy.

Step 6 Understand that your feelings of unhealthy jealousy stem largely from your irrational beliefs about this threat and are not caused by the threat itself

In this book I have emphasized several times that activating events, or critical As to be more precise, contribute to but do not cause your feelings, behaviour and subsequent thinking at point C in the ABCDEFG framework. Rather, how you feel, act and think depends largely (but not exclusively) on the beliefs you hold about these As. Thus, it is important that Darren fully accepts the view that his feelings of unhealthy jealousy about losing the exlusivity of his relationship with Kath (which is, if you recall, an inference) depend on the irrational beliefs he holds about this threat and not on the threat alone.

If you are not convinced that your feelings of unhealthy jealousy are determined largely by irrational beliefs, please re-read Chapter 2.

Step 7 Identify your irrational beliefs and discriminate them from their rational alternatives

After you have fully embraced the view that your feelings of unhealthy jealousy are largely determined by your irrational beliefs, the next step is to identify the specific irrational beliefs that you held in the episode under consideration. As part of this identification process, it is important that you distinguish these irrational beliefs from their rational alternatives. This task is fairly straightforward if you bear in mind the points made in Chapters 2 and 3. You will recall that there are four major irrational beliefs:

- rigid demands
- awfulizing beliefs
- low frustration tolerance beliefs
- depreciation beliefs.

The rational alternatives to these irrational beliefs are as follows:

- full preferences

- anti-awfulizing beliefs
- high frustration tolerance beliefs
- acceptance beliefs.

Let's see how Darren put this information into practice.

First, after he acknowledged that he felt unhealthily jealous about the prospect of losing his exclusive relationship with Kath, Darren looked for his rigid demand which, he realized, lay at the core of his unhealthy jealousy. He showed himself that he did not just prefer not to lose this relationship, he demanded that he must not lose it.

Second, Darren looked for his awfulizing belief. He appreciated that when he felt unhealthily jealous he was not just saying that it would be bad if he lost his exclusive relationship with Kath. He acknowledged that he was making a grossly exaggerated awfulizing statement ('It would be awful if I lost my exclusive relationship with Kath').

Third, Darren looked for and found his LFT belief. He accepted that when he felt unhealthily jealous he was not just saying that losing the exclusive nature of his relationship with Kath would be difficult to bear, but was telling himself, 'I couldn't bear it if I were to lose my exclusive relationship with Kath.'

Finally, Darren looked for his depreciating beliefs and found a self-depreciating belief. He acknowledged that he was not only evaluating the prospect of losing his exclusive relationship with Kath as being bad, but was also saying that this would prove that he was unlovable as a person.

You will find it helpful to use what Darren did as a model for identifying your own irrational beliefs.

Step 8 Challenge these irrational beliefs by showing yourself that they are false, illogical and self-defeating

Now that you have identified the specific irrational beliefs that underpin your feelings of unhealthy jealousy, the next step is to dispute these beliefs. This is the D part of the ABCDEFG framework. The purpose of disputing is to weaken your conviction in your irrational beliefs and to work towards feeling healthily jealous instead. Let me illustrate how you can dispute your irrational beliefs by showing you how Darren disputed his. In doing so, I will focus on Darren's rigid demand and self-depreciation belief. He asked himself and answered the following three questions of his irrational belief:

- Is my irrational belief helpful? Does it give me healthy results?
- Is my irrational belief true? Is it consistent with reality?
- Is my irrational belief sensible or logical?

Darren's irrational belief is: I must not lose my exclusive relationship with Kath. If I do lose this it proves that I am less worthy as a person.

Question: Is this belief helpful?
Answer: No, it is not. This belief will lead me to experience unhealthy jealousy and lead me to behave in a manner that will make it more likely rather than less likely that I will lose my exclusive relationship with Kath and may even lead me to lose her altogether.

Question: Is this belief true?
Answer: Most definitely not. First, if there was a law of the universe that prohibited me from losing my exclusive relationship with Kath, then I could not possibly lose it. Since Kath is a free agent and can choose to have a relationship with whoever she wants, this proves that my demand is not true. Second, if I did lose my exclusive relationship with Kath, it would not prove that I was less worthy as a person. If I have worth as a person it is not dependent on my having an exclusive relationship with Kath. My worth as a person, if it depends on anything, is dependent on my being alive, human and unique. In other words, my worth remains constant during my lifetime.

Question: Is this belief sensible?

Answer: No, it is illogical. I want to have an exclusive relationship with Kath, but this does not prove that I have to have it. What has to be does not follow logically from what I want to happen. Also, while losing my exclusive relationship with Kath is bad, this is just one aspect of my life, and when I conclude that this makes me less worthy as a person, I am making the part-whole error where I say that my entire self can be depreciated on the basis of a part of my life being bad. This is obviously nonsense since it is not possible to rate the whole on the basis of one of its parts.

Using the same three questions, why don't you dispute the irrational beliefs that underpin your situationally based unhealthy jealousy. The effects of disputing your irrational beliefs occur at E in the ABCDEFG framework. The more you challenge your irrational beliefs and really see that they are false, illogical and unhelpful, the healthier these effects at E will be.

Step 9 Show yourself that the rational alternatives to these irrational beliefs, by contrast, are true, sensible and yield healthy results

When you challenge your irrational beliefs, it is akin to uprooting weeds in a garden. However, if your garden is to be full of pretty flowers, you also have to prepare the ground and plant seeds so that these flowers will grow and flourish. Thus, if your rational beliefs are to grow and flourish, then you have to sow them into your belief system. The first step in this process is to apply the same questions to your rational beliefs as you applied to your irrational beliefs in the previous step. Doing this enables you to see clearly why your rational belief is rational and helps you to commit yourself to strengthening your conviction in it and to feel healthy jealousy instead of unhealthy jealousy.

In showing you how this can be done, let's consider how Darren questioned his rational belief which was: 'I don't want to lose my exclusive relationship with Kath, but there is no reason why I must not lose this aspect of my relationship with her. If I do lose this, I am still a worthwhile person even though I have lost something important to me.'

Question: Is this belief helpful?

Answer: Yes, very helpful. It will help me to be concerned and healthily vigilant rather than anxious and hypervigilant. These are features of healthy jealousy as opposed to unhealthy jealousy and encourage me to tell Kath how I feel and check out my hunches with her rather than regard them as facts. I will therefore be unlikely to act in a way that will jeopardize my relationship with Kath.

Question: Is this belief true?

Answer: Yes, it is true. The truth of the matter is that I don't want to lose my exclusive relationship with Kath, but in recognizing that this does not mean that I am immune from losing it, I am acknowledging the reality that this could possibly happen. My belief allows me to accept, but actively dislike, the grim reality that since Kath is a free agent, she can choose to have a relationship with whoever she wants. Second, my belief is true in that if I did lose my exclusive relationship with Kath, I could prove that it would be bad, but that I am still the same fallible human being that I was when I had the exclusive relationship with her. As I said earlier, my worth, if it depends on anything, depends on my being alive, human and unique. In other words, my worth remains constant during my lifetime whether I have an exclusive relationship with Kath or not.

Question: Is this belief sensible?

Answer: Yes, it is sensible. Since I believe that I want to have an exclusive relationship with Kath, it follows logically that I don't have to have one. Basically, what I am saying here is that I don't have to have what I want. This is sensible and contrasts markedly with the statement

84

that I have to have what I want. Also, my conclusion that I am a fallible human being whether or not I have an exclusive relationship with Kath is sensible, since here I am not making the part-whole error which is inherent in the belief that losing my exclusive relationship with Kath diminishes me as a person. My personhood or 'self' is too complex to be rated and even if it could be rated, it is sensible to base this rating on conditions that don't change, like my aliveness, humanity and uniqueness.

Using the same three questions, why don't you question the rational beliefs that underpin your situationally based healthy jealousy. The results of this questioning again occur at E in the ABCDEFG framework. The more convincing your responses to these questions are, the healthier these effects will be.

Step 10 Strengthen your conviction in your rational belief

After you have gained some experience at questioning both your irrational and your rational beliefs, the next step is for you to continue the change process by using techniques that are designed to further weaken your conviction in your irrational belief and to further strengthen your conviction in your rational belief. This part of the process is known as the facilitating change stage and occurs at point F in the ABCDEFG framework. In this section, I will describe two such techniques. These are known as the attack-response technique and the emotive-imagery technique.

The attack-response technique

The purpose of the attack-response technique is for you to gain practice at strengthening your conviction in your rational belief by attacking it with irrational arguments and by responding to these arguments with rational rebuttals until you cannot think of any more irrational arguments.

Here is a set of instructions that I usually give to my clients who I have asked to use this technique.

1 Write down your rational belief on a piece of paper and rate your present level of conviction in this belief next to it using a 100-point scale where 0 = no conviction and 100 = total conviction.
2 Respond to this rational belief with an attack that is directed at this belief. This may take the form of a doubt, reservation or objection to the healthy belief and should be put in the form of an irrational belief. Make this attacking statement as genuinely as you can. The more it reflects what you actually believe, the better. Write down this attack underneath the rational belief.
3 Respond to this attack as fully as you can. It is really important that you respond to each element of the attack. Do so as persuasively as possible and write down this response underneath the first attack.
4 Continue in this vein until you have answered all your attacks and cannot think of any more.

If you find this exercise difficult, you might find it easier to make your attacks gently at first. Then, when you find that you can respond to these attacks quite easily, begin to make the attacks more biting. Work in this way until you are making really strong attacks. When you make an attack, do so as if you want yourself to believe it. And when you respond, really throw yourself into your response with the intention of demolishing the attack and raising your level of conviction in your healthy belief.

Don't forget that the purpose of this exercise is to strengthen your rational belief, so it is important that you stop only when you have answered all your attacks.

When you have answered all your attacks and cannot think of any more, write out your original rational belief and re-rate your level of conviction using the same 100-point scale as before. You should find that your rating has increased.

Here is how Darren used the attack-response technique:

Rational belief: I don't want to lose my exclusive relationship with Kath, but there is no reason why I must not lose this aspect of my relationship with her. If I do lose this, I am still a worthwhile person even though I have lost something important to me.[40]

Attack: But I don't really believe this. I feel as if I really do need an exclusive relationship with Kath.

Response: Of course I don't believe this yet. I need to work hard to convince myself of this. While I may feel that I need an exclusive relationship with Kath, this doesn't meant that it is true. I do want an exclusive relationship with Kath, but that doesn't mean that I have to have one. Just because I really want something doesn't mean that I have to have it.

Attack: But if I don't have an exclusive relationship with Kath, it makes me less worthwhile.

Response: No it doesn't. If I don't have an exclusive relationship with Kath it means that I don't have something that I really want. Not having something that I really want doesn't detract from my worth. I am worthwhile because I am alive, human and unique, not because I have an exclusive relationship with Kath.

Attack: But that's not how most people think. Most people would think that they would be less worthwhile if they lost the exclusive love of someone that they really care about and this means that I'm less worthwhile if this happens to me.

Response: I'm not sure that it is true that most people would think that way. But even if most people do, that doesn't make it sensible. Believing that I am less worthwhile if I don't have an exclusive relationship with Kath isn't sensible because it just doesn't follow. I can rate not having an exclusive relationship with Kath as bad because it is a discrete experience, but rating myself as less worthwhile as a result is based on the idea that I can rate the whole of me on the basis of one experience, which is obviously nonsense.

Rational belief: I don't want to lose my exclusive relationship with Kath, but there is no reason why I must not lose this aspect of my relationship with her. If I do lose this, I am still a worthwhile person even though I have lost something important to me.[75]

The emotive-imagery technique

The second technique that I will describe involves the use of imagery or the pictures that you conjure up in your mind. Don't be concerned if you don't get clear mental pictures; the emotive-imagery technique works whether you get clear images or not. This is how you use the emotive-imagery technique.

1 Identify a specific event at A about which you felt unhealthy jealousy.
2 Close your eyes and vividly imagine this event, focusing on the aspect of the event that you felt most unhealthily jealous about (known as the critical A).
3 Deliberately rehearse the irrational belief that led you to feel unhealthily jealous.
4 Allow yourself really to feel unhealthily jealous while focusing on the critical A in your mind's eye.
5 While still imagining the critical A, change your irrational belief to your rational belief and stay with this new belief until you experience healthy jealousy.
6 Keep with this rational belief and your feelings of healthy

jealousy for about five minutes, all the time imagining the critical part of the event. If you go back to your former irrational belief, bring the rational one back.

7 Practise this technique three times a day for thirty days and see what difference it makes.

Step 11 Act on your new rational belief

One of the best ways of integrating your new rational belief into your belief system is to act on this belief. You need to select those behaviours that would be consistent with your new beliefs. In addition, after you have selected these behaviours, it is important to acknowledge that you need to put them into practice repeatedly if you are going to internalize your new rational belief. I suggest that you re-read Chapter 3, where I discuss behaviours that stem from and are thus consistent with healthy jealousy.

When they got home Darren decided to tell Kath about his feelings of healthy jealousy when he saw Kath laughing and joking with the man at the party. He told her that he loved her very much and was concerned that he might lose her exclusive love. He didn't assume that he would lose the exclusive relationship that he had with her, but checked out with her what the interaction with the man meant to her. This style of interaction didn't put Kath on the defensive. Rather, it enabled her to admit that she was attracted to the man but didn't want any kind of relationship with him. Kath then asked Darren whether he wanted to have a relationship with every woman that he found attractive. Because he felt healthily jealous about this event, Darren saw the power of Kath's argument.

Step 12 Question the thinking consequences of your unhealthy jealousy

In Chapter 2, I discussed how unhealthy jealousy affects the way you subsequently think. At this point, it is important that you stand back and consider how realistic these thoughts are. Feeling healthily jealous rather than unhealthily jealous will help you to be objective as you do this.

89

In Darren's case, his feelings of unhealthy jealousy and the irrational beliefs that underpinned these feelings led him to think the following:

1 'I can't trust Kath again.'
2 'Because Kath is laughing and joking with the man, it means that she finds me boring.'
3 'Kath is looking to begin a relationship with this other man as soon as my back is turned.'
4 'If she is interested in this man, there will be plenty of other men that she is interested in.'

It is important that you question such thoughts, rather than regard them as statements of fact. They are, as you will recognize, inferences that stem from the irrational beliefs that underpin unhealthy jealousy. I recommend that you question these thoughts after, rather than before, you have challenged your rational beliefs, when you can acknowledge that your rational alternative beliefs are true, sensible and helpful. I recommend this order because this type of thinking stems from your irrational beliefs. In other words, they occur at C in the ABCDEFG framework and stem from B, in this case your irrational beliefs.

However, you can, of course, question such thoughts before you challenge your irrational beliefs. Or you might experiment with both orders and see which is more helpful to you. Whichever order you choose, the type of questions you can employ are the same. Here are some examples:

1 How realistic is my thinking here? If it is not realistic, what is a more realistic way of viewing the situation?
2 How likely is it that my inference is true? If it is unlikely to be true, what inference is most likely to be true?
3 Would 12 objective judges agree that my inference is correct? If not, what would they conclude is most likely to be true?
4 If I asked someone whom I could trust to give me an objective opinion about the truth or falsity of my inference, what would this person say to me and why? How would this person encourage me to view the situation instead?

5 If someone told me that they had made this inference about the same situation, what would I say to this person about the validity of their inference and why? How would I encourage the person to view the situation instead?
6 What data do I need to gather to check the validity of my inference, and how reliable will such data be?

When your thinking is coloured by unhealthy jealousy, much of your thoughts will be about your partner and your relationship. As such, it is worthwhile thinking about your partner and your relationship when you are not feeling unhealthily jealous, and making a written response to the following illustrative questions:

1 From what I know about my partner, what evidence do I have that
  • she will . . . (e.g. wish to go off with the first attractive man that she encounters)?
  • she will not . . . (e.g. wish to go off with the first attractive man that she encounters)?
2 From what I know of my relationship with my partner, what evidence do I have that
  • this relationship is not . . . (e.g. solid)?
  • this relationship is . . . (e.g. solid)?

The more you can think realistically about your partner and your relationship when you are not feeling unhealthily jealous, the more you will be able to do so once you have experienced unhealthy jealousy about a specific event and challenged the irrational beliefs that underpinned these feelings.

Step 13 Reconsider the nature of the threat to your relationship

You will recall that in Step 5 I asked you to identify what you felt most unhealthily jealous about in the episode that you chose to analyse. I also urged you to assume temporarily that the threat to your relationship was real. I encouraged you to do this to identify the irrational beliefs that lay at the core of your feelings of unhealthy jealousy. If you had checked to see whether or not your relationship with your partner was really under threat at this point you might have stopped feeling unhealthily jealous, but you would have achieved this without identifying, challenging and changing the irrational beliefs tht really determined your feelings of unhealthy jealousy. In REBT, we call this changing A rather than changing B. If you had bypassed your irrational beliefs at this point, you would still be vulnerable to feeling unhealthily jealous about the event in question if you later thought that you had been correct in the first place and that your relationship was actually under threat. In addition, if you had challenged your critical A without first challenging your irrational beliefs, your challenge of your critical A would have been coloured by the ongoing existence of these irrational beliefs.

You are in a much better position, therefore, to question your critical A that your relationship is under threat in some way after you have challenged and changed your irrational beliefs. Doing so will help you to be objective in your questioning of your critical A. Putting this differently, feeling healthily jealous will help you to stand back and take an objective view about your critical inference at A, while feeling unhealthily jealous will interfere with your objectivity. When you come to evaluate whether or not your relationship with your partner was under threat in the episode under consideration, why not ask yourself the questions that I outlined in Step 12 above?

> Feeling healthily jealous rather than unhealthily jealous in the episode that he chose to analyse helped Darren to be objective about his inference that he was losing the exclusive relationship that he had with Kath as a result of her laughing and joking with the man at the party. On thinking about this issue, but this time from a more objective position, Darren concluded (with the help of similar questions to those that I detailed on pp. 90–91) that while he didn't like Kath's behaviour, it indicated that she was being friendly with the man, and did not prove that she was interested in forming a relationship with him in addition to the relationship she had with Darren.

In this chapter, I have discussed the 13 steps that you need to take to overcome your feelings of situationally based unhealthy jealousy. In the next and final chapter, I will offer you some guidance about what you need to do in order to become less prone to unhealthy jealousy.

5

Twenty Ways To Become Less Prone to Unhealthy Jealousy

I have written this chapter especially for those who are particularly prone to unhealthy jealousy and who wish to become less prone to this destructive emotion. If you are in any doubt whether or not you are prone to experience unhealthy jealousy, I suggest that you re-read pp. 40–46. So what can you do to make yourself less prone to what some have called the green-eyed monster? By putting into practice the following 20 suggestions.

Take responsibility for being prone to unhealthy jealousy

It is very important that you take responsibility for being prone to unhealthy jealousy. You may think that your partner makes you feel unhealthily jealous by her behaviour, but this is not the case even if your partner does overtly flirt with other men. No, while your partner's behaviour does contribute to how you feel, you largely make yourself unhealthily jealous by the irrational beliefs that you hold about her behaviour. Unless you accept this point you will not actively look for, challenge and change your irrational beliefs and may well continue to blame your partner for your feelings, in which case you will perpetuate your proneness to experience unhealthy jealousy. However, if you do accept responsibility for your unhealthy jealousy, you will have taken the important step in helping yourself to become less prone to experiencing this destructive emotion.

Acknowledge that unhealthy jealousy is a problem for you

Once you have acknowledged that you are responsible for making yourself unhealthily jealous, the next step is for you to acknowledge fully that this form of jealousy is a problem for you. Take a sheet of paper and write down the advantages and disadvantages of experiencing unhealthy jealousy, both from a short-term and from a long-term perspective. Review times when you have experienced unhealthy jealousy and remember what were the consequences of this emotion. You might find it helpful to re-read Chapter 2 before you do so. If you do this exercise conscientiously, then, in all probability, you will see that the disadvantages of experiencing unhealthy jealousy clearly outweigh any advantages.

Once you have listed the advantages and disadvantages of unhealthy jealousy, you might find it helpful to question whether or not the advantages really are benefits. For example, if you said that unhealthy jealousy is a sign that you really care for your partner, question this statement and show yourself that this form of jealousy is a sign of disturbance rather than a sign of caring for your partner. Continue questioning what you consider to be the positive aspects of your unhealthy jealousy until you have acknowledged that most are really negative.

Acknowledge that healthy jealousy is the healthy alternative to unhealthy jealousy

Before you take this step review Chapter 3, which is devoted to outlining the nature of healthy jealousy. Then, when you are clear that you have understood why this type of jealousy is healthy, take another sheet of paper and write down the advantages and disadvantages of experiencing healthy jealousy, again from both a short-term and a long-term perspective. Review those same occasions when you experienced unhealthy jealousy, but this time imagine that you experienced healthy jealousy instead. Focus on what would have been the consequences of this alternative emotion.

The next step is to list the advantages and disadvantages of healthy jealousy in the same way as you did for unhealthy jealousy. Once you have done this you will be able to see that the advantages of healthy jealousy far outweigh its disadvantages. Indeed, you will find it helpful to question whether or not the disadvantages of healthy jealousy are really disadvantages.

Commit yourself to becoming healthily jealous

After you have fully understood that healthy jealousy is the constructive alternative to unhealthy jealousy, make a commitment to work towards experiencing this emotion when you face, or think that you face, threats to your relationship. You might find it helpful to make a written commitment to yourself and review this every day. Also, you might like to make a verbal commitment to a close friend with whom you might discuss your progress over the coming weeks and months.

Accept yourself for being prone to unhealthy jealousy

Once you have taken responsibility for largely creating your feelings of unhealthy jealousy, acknowledged that you are prone to experiencing this emotion and that it is a problem for you, can clearly see that healthy jealousy is an acceptable alternative for you to work towards and have made a commitment to do so, you need then to accept yourself for being so prone if in fact you put yourself down for having a jealousy problem. This involves realizing that you are an unrateable, complex individual who is constantly in flux, and that you have positive, neutral and negative aspects, one of which is your propensity to make yourself unhealthily jealous, a propensity that you can work on and largely overcome, albeit not perfectly.

When you depreciate yourself for being prone to experiencing unhealthy jealousy, you rate your entire 'self' on the basis of this proneness. Making a global rating of yourself serves only to distract you from working to overcome your jealousy problem, whereas accepting yourself for having this problem enables you to devote your resources to addressing the problem. So, if you depreciate yourself for being particularly prone to unhealthy jealousy, work on accepting yourself for having this problem before you address it directly. You can use the disputing methods that I outlined on pp. **81–83** to help you to do this.

Keep working on specific episodes of unhealthy jealousy

In the previous chapter, I outlined the steps that you need to take when working on specific episodes of unhealthy jealousy. In particular, I showed you how to identify what you were most unhealthily jealous about and how to assess, challenge and change the irrational beliefs that underpinned your situationally based unhealthy jealousy. I recommend that, as soon as you begin to notice that you are making yourself unhealthily jealous, you follow the steps that I have delineated in the previous chapter. Initially, you will need to do this on paper, but after much practice you will be able to do it in your head. You will also be able to anticipate situations in which you may make yourself unhealthily jealous and deal productively with these situations before they actually occur.

I do need to stress to you that in order for you to be able to overcome your feelings of unhealthy jealousy by identifying, challenging and changing your irrational beliefs in your head, both when you begin to experience this destructive emotion in actual situations and before you enter such situations, you will have to put in a lot of written practice of working through specific episodes of situationally based unhealthy jealousy. However, if you do this diligently you will develop your skills at overcoming situationally based unhealthy jealousy, and as you do so you will begin to become generally less prone to the green-eyed monster.

Identify the themes in your specific examples of unhealthy jealousy

Once you have worked through a number of specific examples of your unhealthy jealousy, you will be able to identify a specific theme or themes which span these examples. These themes occur at A in the ABCDEFG framework. In other words, they are general types of situations about which you make yourself jealous. It is important that you fully appreciate that these themes contribute to your feelings of unhealthy jealousy, rather than directly causing these feelings. Remember that it is your irrational beliefs about these themes that are at the core of your proneness to experience unhealthy jealousy, rather than the themes themselves.

When you have identified the themes that span the specific examples of your unhealthy jealousy, I suggest that you make a written note of them, since they will come in handy when you come to identify the general irrational beliefs that help to explain why you are so prone to unhealthy jealousy. In Chapter 4, I argued that typical themes in unhealthy jealousy concern:

- losing your relationship with your partner;
- losing the exclusive nature of your relationship with your partner;
- losing your place as the most important person in your partner's life;
- having other people of the same sex as you show an interest in your partner.

You might find it helpful to bear these themes in mind as you strive to identify the major theme or themes that are present in your own experience of unhealthy jealousy.

Identify, challenge and change your general irrational beliefs

After you have identified the major theme or themes that recur at A in the ABCDEFG framework, you are ready to identify, challenge and change the general irrational beliefs that are at the core of your proneness to experience unhealthy jealousy. Let me give you some common examples of such general irrational beliefs.

1 I must not lose my relationship with my partner. If I did, it would be awful and unbearable and it would prove that I am a nobody.
2 I must have an exclusive relationship with my partner. It would be terrible if I lost this exclusivity and my life would be intolerable if that happened. It would also prove that I am unlovable.
3 I must at all times be the most important person in my partner's life, and it would be horrendous if I wasn't. Losing this status would be too much to bear and would prove that I was less worthy than the person who has replaced me in my partner's affections.
4 I must be the only man in my partner's life, and this means that other men must not show any interest in her at all. If they do it would be the end of the world and I couldn't stand it. They would be rotten people for doing what I decree that they must not do.
5 I must know at all times that my relationship with my partner is not under threat. It would be awful if I did not have such knowledge, and not being certain means that my relationship is under threat.

The above are general irrational beliefs in that they are not related to specific activating events at A in the ABCDEFG framework. They will, however, be manifest in these specific events. Thus, if you hold the last general irrational belief that I outlined above and you encounter a specific example of uncertainty, then you will hold a specific irrational belief, such as: 'I saw Jane speaking to Harry in the bar. I must know for sure that their conversation was innocent and it will be terrible if I don't know this. Not knowing means that it wasn't innocent.'

You challenge your general irrational beliefs in the same way as you learned to challenge your specific irrational beliefs. Thus, you take one of your general irrational beliefs and ask yourself and answer the following questions:

- Is this belief true?
- Is this belief logical?
- Is this belief helpful?

At this point, you might find it beneficial to review the material on disputing specific irrational beliefs that I covered on pp. 81–83.

Next, you need to develop rational alternatives to these general irrational beliefs, and once you have done this you need to question these general rational beliefs in the same way as you questioned your general irrational beliefs. Do this until you can see clearly that your general rational beliefs are true, sensible and helpful and that your general irrational beliefs are, by contrast, false, illogical and unhelpful. The effects that you derive occur at E in the ABCDEFG framework and will be healthier the more convincing you find the answers to your questions.

Then, I suggest that you use the attack-response technique to deepen your conviction in your general rational belief (see pp. 85–88 for a reminder of how to use this technique). This technique is an example of the facilitating change which occurs at F in the ABCDEFG framework.

Accept yourself even if your relationship really is under threat

In my experience as a counsellor working with people who are prone to unhealthy jealousy, it is clear that at bottom such people have low self-esteem. They generally regard themselves as unworthy, unlovable individuals who have very little to offer potential partners. Once they have developed a relationship with a person, their stance to that relationship is twofold. First, they believe that they need the relationship to prove to themselves that they are not unworthy; on the other hand, because they believe that they are unworthy, they cannot convince themselves that their partners will stay with them in the face of opposition from potential rivals. The more deeply a person believes that he will not be able to compete with such competition, the more he will see other men as threats to his relationship with his partner and the more he will see other men as rivals.

It follows from this that if you are to become less prone to unhealthy jealousy, it is very important that you develop a healthy attitude towards yourself. This subject warrants a book on its own, and indeed my colleague, Dr Paul Hauck, has written such a book, entitled *Hold Your Head Up High* (Sheldon Press, 1991). I recommend that you read this book and apply Dr Hauck's innovative methods. What I will do here is outline briefly some of the issues that you need to consider if you are to develop a healthy attitude to yourself, which is best described as unconditional self-acceptance.

1 Recognize that your 'self' is incredibly complex and comprises all the thoughts, emotions, behaviours, images and sensations that you have experienced or enacted from the day you were born until the moment you die. It also includes all your bodily aspects and personality characteristics. As such it is far too complex to be given a global rating, although parts of your 'self' can be rated.
2 Rather than rate yourself, it is more healthy for you to accept yourself unconditionally.
3 Recognize that if you have an essence as a human being it is that you are fallible and unique.
4 Realize that as a person you are no better and no worse than other humans, although you are unequal to others in many different specific respects.

5 Appreciate that when you accept yourself you think logically and avoid making overgeneralization errors.

6 Unconditional self-acceptance rests on a philosophy of flexible, full preferences. So strive to think flexibly and avoid making rigid demands of yourself and other people.

7 Note that when you accept yourself, your emotions are healthy and your behaviour is constructive. Self-acceptance does not, therefore, promote indifference or resignation.

8 If you still want to rate yourself, judge yourself against conditions that do not change in your lifetime. Thus, think of yourself as worthwhile because you are human, alive and unique, and not because your partner loves you, for example.

9 You can learn to accept yourself unconditionally, but you cannot do so perfectly, nor for all time.

10 Internalizing a philosophy of unconditional self-acceptance is difficult and involves hard work and work that is active and forceful.

Develop a healthy attitude about relationships

People who are prone to unhealthy jealousy generally have an unhealthy attitude about relationships. Some, as I pointed out above, see their relationship with their partner as essential to them being able to sustain a view of themselves as worthy, lovable individuals. Others see their partner as their property and believe that the other person's main function is to behave according to their wishes. As you may be able to tell, both of these stances are unlikely to lead to stable, fulfilling relationships. In the first case, your partner is likely to find the job of making you feel good about yourself wearing and onerous after a while, and in the second case, your partner will soon become fed up with your attempts to possess her.

Whether you attempt to use your relationship with your partner as a regulator of your self-esteem or whether you attempt to possess your partner, the behaviours you employ to achieve your ends only serve to make it more rather than less likely that your partner will leave you. This is known as a self-fulfilling prophecy.

This is how the self-fulfilling prophecy in unhealthy jealousy works. First, you begin by doubting that your partner really loves you and believing that he will eventually leave you. Second, your behaviour is influenced by your resultant unhealthy jealousy and insecurity. Third, your behaviour has a negative impact on your partner and eventually he leaves you for someone else. Finally, you conclude that you were correct all along: potential partners will end up leaving you for someone else, a conclusion or rule which you take to your next relationship, and the entire sequence gets played out again.

You will note from my description of the self-fulfilling prophecy in unhealthy jealousy that nowhere is there an acknowledgment that you take responsibility for helping to bring about the end of your relationship with your partner. Rather, you portray yourself as a victim. The only way that you can break the vicious circle of unhealthy jealousy self-fulfilling prophecy is to take responsibility for your behaviour, acknowledge the impact that this has had on successive partners and identify, challenge and change the specific and general irrational beliefs that underpin your behaviour.

Develop a healthy attitude towards uncertainty and not knowing

If you are prone to unhealthy jealousy, it is very likely that you have an unhealthy attitude towards uncertainty about whether or not your partner is interested in someone else. In addition, you also probably have an unhealthy attitude towards not knowing what your partner is doing and with whom she is doing it. Because you believe that you must be certain that your partner is not interested in someone else, and you think that it is terrible to be faced with such uncertainty, you tend to think that if you are uncertain about this issue then your partner really is interested in another person. If you can't convince yourself that she is not interested in a rival, then, faced with a choice between living with the uncertainty and concluding that she is interested in a third person, your unhealthy attitude towards uncertainty and your other irrational beliefs that underpin your unhealthy jealousy will lead you to think the latter.

Similarly, if you do not know who your partner is with and what she is doing, your intolerance about not knowing and your other unhealthy jealousy-related irrational beliefs will lead you to be very suspicious of your partner and think that what she is doing constitutes a threat to your relationship.

If you wish to become less prone to unhealthy jealousy, it is very important that you develop a healthy attitude to uncertainty and not knowing. This involves challenging your demanding beliefs about uncertainty and recognizing that while you prefer to have certainty about absence of threat to your relationship with your partner, for example, you do not need to have such certainty. Realize that while uncertainty and not knowing are difficult to put up with, they are definitely tolerable.

Also, it is important to recognize that when you demand certainty, this demand leads you to overestimate threat to your relationship when you are uncertain. However, if you give up this demand but remain with your healthy preference for certainty, then you will not equate uncertainty with threat. So, it is really important for you to acknowledge that, when you demand certainty and knowledge and you act on these demands, you serve only to perpetuate and deepen your proneness to experience unhealthy jealousy. By contrast, if you challenge and change these demands and remain with your preferences for knowledge and certainty, you will be more flexible about when to act to attempt to gain more certainty and better knowledge and when to do nothing. In addition, you will be much more likely to give your partner the benefit of the doubt and will begin to trust him more.

Develop a healthy attitude to not being in control and not having what you want

One of the problems of people who are prone to unhealthy jealousy is a dogmatic attitude about being in control of their relationships. This frequently manifests itself in a demand that they must have control over their partner. If you have such a belief, it is very likely that you insist that your partner does what you want when you want her to do it, and this becomes heightened when your partner understandably wants time for herself to see her friends, pursue her hobbies and generally be a person in her own right. If you have a dire need to be in charge, then you will be highly threatened by these perfectly natural and healthy human desires. Indeed, because you are intolerant of her desires, you will tend to view them as evidence that she is fed up with you, doesn't love you any more and will use these periods away from you as opportunities to meet a new partner. This is why a dire need to be in charge and in control, as well as an insistence that your partner must do what you want her to do, is centrally involved in the possessive type of unhealthy jealousy.

If you want to be less prone to unhealthy jealousy, it follows that you need to internalize and act on a healthy philosophy towards being in control in your relationship with your partner and with respect to getting what you want from her. Thus, it is important for you to recognize that while there may be advantages to being in control in your relationship, this does not have to be its essential feature. Indeed, the more you allow your partner autonomy, the healthier your relationship with her will be. Also, you need to appreciate that getting what you want is fine, but when you transform this desire into a rigid must, you deprive your partner of getting a share of what she wants in life. As a result, she will become dissatisfied and tend to pull away from you, something which you definitely do not want to happen. So, strike a balance between getting what you want and encouraging – yes, encouraging – your partner to get what she wants from life. If you do so, you will become less prone to unhealthy jealousy and will have a better relationship with your partner as a consequence.

Accept your partner if she acts in ways in which you disapprove

As I mentioned in Chapter 2, unhealthy anger towards your partner can be a major feature of unhealthy jealousy, either when you experience this emotion situationally or when you are highly prone to experience it. If unhealthy anger towards your partner is a feature of your proneness to experience unhealthy jealousy, it is important that you address it if you are to become less prone to the green-eyed monster.

This involves developing an attitude of acceptance when your partner acts in ways that you dislike and that go against your preferences. In this context, acceptance does not mean resignation, nor does it mean condoning actions of which you disapprove. It acknowledges that your partner is a fallible human being who acts well and badly and cannot be defined by her actions. So, while it makes sense for you to rate negatively what your partner does when this is against your preferences, it does not make sense to rate her negatively as a result. Also, accepting your partner means ensuring that you don't transform your healthy, flexible preferences concerning her behaviour into rigid demands. If you develop and maintain such an accepting attitude towards your partner, you will still experience anger when your partner acts against your wishes, but this type of anger will be healthy and promote a constructive dialogue between your partner and yourself. It is also closely related to healthy jealousy which, as discussed in Chapter 3, is the healthy alternative to unhealthy jealousy. If unhealthy anger is a major feature of your unhealthy jealousy, you might find it useful to consult my book on the subject, entitled *Overcoming Anger: When Anger Helps and When it Hurts* (Sheldon Press, 1996).

Appreciate that your general irrational beliefs lead you to overestimate threats to your relationship with your partner

I am often asked why people who are particularly prone to unhealthy jealousy see something as a threat to their relationship, when other people who face exactly the same situation do not see it as threatening in that respect. For example, you and your friend may see your respective spouses laughing and joking with another man at a party, but why do you think that your partner wants to start a relationship with the man whereas your friend is pleased that his wife is enjoying herself? In my opinion, the answer lies in the different beliefs held by people who are prone to unhealthy jealousy and those who are not thus prone. This means that when you are particularly prone to experience unhealthy jealousy you bring your set of general irrational beliefs to events, and these beliefs influence the type of inferences that you make about these situations. Thus, if you hold the following general irrational belief: 'My partner must not show any interest in another woman and it would be awful if he did', and you see him talking with interest to a woman at a social gathering, your general irrational belief will lead you to overestimate the threat to your relationship posed by this incident.

If your partner is doing something that you believe he is not supposed to be doing, then this rigid extreme belief will mean that it is more likely that you will think he fancies her than if you held a general rational belief such as: 'I would prefer it if my partner does not show interest in another woman but there is certainly no reason why he must not do so. If he did it would be bad, but not awful.'

If you can see the influence that your general irrational beliefs at B have on the inferences that you make at A, then you will be more likely to search for and challenge these beliefs than if you do not see this influence. If you lack this insight you will become preoccupied with the events at A, whereas if you have this insight you will go to the source of your unhealthy jealousy – namely your irrational beliefs – and work at that source. In doing so, you will become less prone to the green-eyed monster.

Identify the action and thinking tendencies associated with your unhealthy jealousy and develop a list of alternative healthy action and thinking tendencies based on your general healthy jealousy-related rational beliefs. Resolve to practise the latter and limit the former

In Chapter 2, I showed you that once you have made yourself unhealthily jealous by holding a set of irrational beliefs about an actual or perceived threat to your relationship, you will tend to act and think in certain ways that are consistent with your unhealthy jealousy. Once you have developed and strengthened your alternative rational beliefs it is very important that you do not unwittingly reinforce your irrational beliefs by acting in ways that are consistent with them. If you do the latter, you will undermine all the good work you have achieved through challenging and changing your specific and general irrational beliefs. What do you need to do instead? My advice is to follow these suggestions.

1 Make a note of the way you act and 'feel' like acting once you feel unhealthily jealous.
2 Develop a list of alternative constructive behaviours that you can carry out instead.
3 Make a note of the way you think once you feel unhealthily jealous.

4 Develop a list of alternative thoughts that you can think instead.
5 After you have identified, challenged and changed your general irrational beliefs and have begun to practise thinking according to your new general rational beliefs, resist strongly the temptation to act and think according to your irrational beliefs. This will be difficult, because you are used to acting and thinking in ways that are consistent with your feelings of unhealthy jealousy. However, if you show yourself that it is worth holding back on these habitual ways of thinking and acting and that you can tolerate the discomfort of so doing, you will help yourself to follow the next step.
6 Resolve to act and think in ways that are consistent with your developing rational beliefs and your new feelings of healthy jealousy, and which you identified in points 2 and 4 above. Accept the fact that you will feel awkward in doing so because you are not used to acting and thinking in these constructive ways. Again, tolerate this discomfort and show yourself that it is worth tolerating. The more you act and think in these more constructive ways, the more used to them you will become.
7 Recognize that, because your old ways of acting and thinking associated with your proneness to feel unhealthily jealous are more habitual than your constructive alternatives, you may well slip back into these old ways. Don't disturb yourself about this, because it is to be expected. Once this happens use your slipping back as a cue both to reassert your general rational beliefs and to return to the newer ways of acting and thinking that are consistent with these rational beliefs.

Making your thoughts and your behaviour consistent with your general rational beliefs is perhaps the best way of facilitating change (F in the ABCDEFG framework).

Identify the threats to which you are particularly sensitive and think objectively about them

As you work towards becoming less prone to unhealthy jealousy, it is important that you become aware of the threats to which you are particularly sensitive. In Chapter 4, I argued that there are four major threats to your relationship that you are likely to feel unhealthily jealous about. These are:

- losing your relationship with your partner;
- losing the exclusive nature of your relationship with your partner;
- losing your place as the most important person in your partner's life;
- having other people of the same sex as you show an interest in your partner.

Earlier on in this chapter, I argued that it was important for you to use these themes when identifying your general irrational beliefs. At this point, I suggest that you stand back and think objectively about them. Thus, you can ask yourself such questions as:

1 How likely is it that I am about to lose my place as the most important person in my partner's life?
2 Would 12 objective observers who have access to all relevant information think I was about to lose my place as the most important person in my partner's life?
3 If a good friend was facing exactly the same situation as me and I was able to think objectively about his situation, would I think that he was about to lose his place as the most important person in his partner's life?

If, in response to such questions, you do not think that the threat is real, then it is important that you arrive at a more accurate inference. If, however, you still think that you are facing this threat, then it is important that you think rationally about it and then take steps to discuss your suspicions with your partner and/or deal with the situation constructively.

Modify the rules that are related to your unhealthy jealousy

In Chapter 2, I argued that when you are unhealthily jealous you have one or more rules that predispose you to unhealthy jealousy. It is important that you become aware of these rules and modify them if you are to become less prone to unhealthy jealousy. The best time to do this is when you have made good progress in relinquishing your general irrational beliefs and in strengthening your conviction in your general rational beliefs. In modifying a rule, ask yourself how consistent it is with all the objective evidence at your disposal (i.e. how true it is); if it is false, write down a rule which you think is more consistent with the evidence and with reality. In doing this exercise, be as objective as you can and write down all the reasons in favour of and against both sets of rules. If you do this exercise while holding your general rational beliefs and while you are in an objective frame of mind, you will probably see that your realistic rule accounts better for the evidence than your unhealthy jealousy rule.

Here are a number of rules that predispose people to unhealthy jealousy and their more realistic alternatives:

Unhealthy jealousy rule: My partner cannot be trusted with other men.
Realistic rule: My partner can basically be trusted with other men unless I have clear-cut evidence to the contrary.

Unhealthy jealousy rule: My partner does not find me attractive, lovable and/or interesting and is bound to find other men more attractive, lovable and/or more interesting than me.
Realistic rule: My partner finds me attractive, lovable and/or interesting and if she finds other men attractive and interesting, she will still find me more attractive and interesting than the other person unless I have clear-cut evidence to the contrary.

Unhealthy jealousy rule: My partner is bound to reject me, betray me or make a fool of me.
Realistic rule: My partner will not reject me, betray me or make a fool of me unless I have clear-cut evidence that this is very likely to happen.

Unhealthy jealousy rule: I have far less to offer my partner than other men do.

Realistic rule: I have at least as much and probably more to offer my partner than other men do.

Unhealthy jealousy rule: All men are predatory and are bound to try to steal my partner away from me.
Realistic rule: Some men (but by no means all) are predatory and some may try to steal my partner away from me.

Finally, it is important that you practise your realistic rules as frequently as possible until you become used to them.

Take an objective view of your partners (both past and present)

When you are unhealthily jealous, you are very likely to have a distorted view of your partners, both past and present. Your jealousy leads you to think of your partners as people who have or who had an eye for the opposite sex and will use any opportunity to become involved with them romantically and/or sexually. Once you have made good progress in overcoming your general irrational beliefs and in strengthening your conviction in your alternative general rational beliefs, you are ready to adopt an objective view of your past and present partners.

Once you are clear about the nature of the threat which you think is posed to your present relationship and the threats that you think occurred to your past relationships, it is important that you consider carefully and objectively how accurate your views were and are of these significant others.

Ask yourself the following question: 'From what I know about the partners that I have had, what evidence do I have that they were the kind of people who wanted to go off with the first attractive person that they encountered?'

Write down such evidence and ask yourself whether it would stand up in a court of law. In law, evidence has to be corroborated independently. Your partners cannot be found guilty, as it were, by you thinking that they are guilty. What would a jury of 12 independent people make of the evidence that you have amassed against your partners? Would they convict your partners on this evidence or would they conclude that your evidence was coloured

110

by your general irrational belefs and the feelings of unhealthy jealousy that these beliefs have given rise to?

After you have made an objective appraisal of your partners (and in most cases, but not all, you will conclude that your view of your partners has been determined by your unhealthy jealousy and is not an accurate reflection of what they are like), give them the benefit of the doubt. This means, for example, that you will need to remind yourself that your partners have probably not been interested in every member of the opposite sex that they have encountered, and even if they have found some of them attractive this does not mean that they have preferred them to you. Do you want to start a relationship with every member of the opposite sex that you find attractive? That is unlikely. If it is true, however, you may be projecting your thoughts of infidelity on to your partners. Just because you may want to be unfaithful doesn't mean that your partners have had similar desires. So, accept the fact that you can't be certain about what your partners have felt about members of the opposite sex; assume that they are innocent until proven guilty rather than guilty until proven innocent, which is how you have viewed your partners in the past and are in danger of viewing your present and future partners unless you choose to do otherwise. The worst thing that can happen is that you trust your partner to be faithful and they prove not to be worthy of your trust. If this happens show yourself that this is a bad state of affairs, but is hardly the end of the world.

So, in a nutshell, my view on this point is as follows: assume that the people that you have been involved with, are currently involved with and may be involved with in the future, are worthy of your trust, and treat them accordingly. Do this and you will become less prone to unhealthy jealousy. Can I give you a guarantee that you will always be right? No, of course not. But you will be correct most of the time. What more can you ask for?

Accept that you can have a good relationship with many people

At the bottom of some people's proneness to unhealthy jealousy is the idea that they can only have a good relationship with a small number of people. If you hold such an idea, it will increase the likelihood that you will believe that you have to make the relationship with your present partner work. In turn, this irrational belief will make you insecure and increase your tendency to view threats to your relationship.

One way of tackling this idea is to show yourself that in all likelihood there are many people in the world that you could have a good relationship with. Realizing this will help you to see that it is desirable but not essential for your relationship with your partner to work. This rational belief will lead you to be more secure and will in turn encourage you to make realistic appraisals of threat to your current relationship. In doing so you will become less prone to unhealthy jealousy.

Learn about the familiarity principle and strive to go against it

The final tip that I want to give you to help you become less prone to unhealthy jealousy involves learning about the familiarity principle of human behaviour as applied to unhealthy jealousy.

The familiarity principle describes a tendency for humans to think, feel and act in ways that are familiar to them and to seek out situations and relationships that are familiar to them as well. Thus, if you are prone to unhealthy jealousy you will find the feelings, thoughts and behaviours that are involved in your jealousy problem familiar and very easy to experience, even though they are destructive to your well-being and to your relationships. Thus, in order for you to become less prone to unhealthy jealousy you will have to tolerate the discomfort of thinking, feeling and acting in ways that are unfamiliar to you.

In addition, you may be puzzled by some of your actions which seem to sabotage your attempts to become less prone to unhealthy jealousy.

For example, one of my clients, Jim, was making good progress at becoming less prone to unhealthy jealousy when one day he astounded himself by introducing his wife to Graham, the office Romeo, at his works Christmas party. Indeed, he did so at a time when the mistletoe was going round and promptly left them alone. When he returned he saw Graham kissing his wife, and predictably he felt unhealthily jealous about this. What Jim was doing here was unconsciously setting up a scenario in which it was likely that he would experience the painful but familiar feelings of unhealthy jealousy. Once I explained the familiarity principle to Jim he saw in a flash what he was doing and admitted to feeling uneasy with his new set of general rational beliefs. In his own words, he didn't feel like himself with these new beliefs and, however painful it was to see his wife kissing Graham, at least he felt like his old familiar self.

If you are working hard to become less prone to unhealthy jealousy using the methods outlined in this book, do appreciate that for a good while you will be uncomfortable thinking, feeling and acting in healthy ways. Please accept the discomfort that is almost always associated with personal change, and if you find yourself setting up situations that make it likely that you will experience your old familiar feelings of unhealthy jealousy, realize that you are operating according to the familiarity principle. Understanding and learning from what you are doing and renewing your resolve to tolerate the unfamiliarity of personal change will help you to transcend the familiarity principle until you become used to experiencing healthy jealousy. In doing so you will become less prone to the green-eyed monster.

This marks the end of the book. I hope that you have found it of some use to you and, as is my custom, I invite your feedback c/o Sheldon Press. Thank you for your attention and interest.

Index